Mini Habits for Weight Loss

Stop Dieting. Form New Habits. Change Your Lifestyle Without Suffering.

By
Stephen Guise

Blog: http://stephenguise.com

Book site: http://minihabits.com

Copyright
Mini Habits for Weight Loss by Stephen Guise

Legal Disclaimer

More From Stephen

Check out **minihabits.com** for additional *Mini Habits for Weight Loss* content, tools, and resources!

Mini Habits
If you haven't yet, I strongly recommend you read my first book, *Mini Habits*. Although you don't need to read *Mini Habits* to benefit from *Mini Habits for Weight Loss*, it will give you more of the nuts and bolts of the original mini habits strategy.

Based on the science, *Mini Habits* is arguably the most effective habit formation strategy in the world. And, based on reviews, it's arguably the most loved and the most successful! Many lives have been transformed as a result of adopting the mini habits strategy. It can change your life too!

Mini Habits book: **http://amazon.com/dp/B00HGKNBDK**

Mini Habit Mastery
If you prefer video and want to learn the mini habits concept, you can take the Mini Habit Mastery Video Course. Use coupon code "MHWL55" for an exclusive *Mini Habits for Weight Loss* discount. Mini Habit Mastery is among the world's most popular habit courses, with over 9,000 students.

Mini Habit Mastery HD Video Course: **https://www.udemy.com/mini-habit-mastery/?couponCode=MHWL55**

How to Be an Imperfectionist
My second book applies *Mini Habits* to the problem of perfectionism. If you struggle with depression, fear, and inaction, this book has a lot to offer. It's the highest-rated product I've ever created.

How to Be an Imperfectionist book: **https://www.amazon.com/dp/B00UMG535Y**

Tuesday Messages
Every Tuesday, I write about smart life strategies and email them to subscribers. People have told me this content is life-changing. When you

sign up, you can look through the archives of previous messages of interest. These are exclusive to subscribers and free. Also, signing up means you'll get to know when my next book or course is available.

Tuesday email sign-up: **http://stephenguise.com/subscribe/**

Table of Contents

Preface

Mini Habits and the One Push-up Story

"Success is simple. Do what's right, the right way, at the right time."
~ Arnold H. Glasow

December 28, 2012

I prefer to do the easiest and most enjoyable things, even if it's sometimes at the expense of moving my life in a healthy direction, and I don't think I'm alone in that.

For most of my life, my propensity to do the fun but less advisable things was extremely frustrating. It kept me from becoming the person I wanted to be. But I found a way to turn the odds in my favor. Not to be dramatic or anything, but my life changed forever on December 28, 2012. Here's what happened.

The end of the year was three days away, and I sat on my bed thinking about making some changes. Namely, I desired to exercise consistently, something I had never been able to do. I'd do it for a week or two and quit. The reasons varied; there was always an excuse.

I'm not fond of New Year's Resolutions with their arbitrary start date of January 1, so I decided to begin my change that day by exercising for 30 minutes at home. Problem: I couldn't do it. I felt lethargic, unmotivated, and out of shape. The idea of exercising actually *repulsed* me, and no motivational tactic helped. I had been in this situation before, but a recent book I read gave me an idea.

Earlier that month, I had read *Thinkertoys* by Michael Michalko. Michalko gives readers a number of creative problem solving tools, one of which is called "False Faces." To use this technique, you simply consider the opposite of your current idea. A crude example: If your idea is to build a water park, maybe the opposite idea would be to build a desert-themed park. The opposite idea is not meant to be great in itself, but to open your mind to a wider spectrum of possibilities.

My idea was to exercise for 30 minutes, but I had hit a motivational brick wall, so I tried out "False Faces" to see if it could solve my problem. Since I saw my workout as an intimidating amount of effort, I figured the opposite would be something that's very easy to do, say, one push-up.

I laughed at myself for considering such a worthless idea.

Thanks for nothing, Mr. Michalko! Your little technique didn't work!

One push-up? I may have been down, but I could do better than that. Eventually, I decided to do it out of self-mockery and frustration for failing to get motivated.

If I can't do a simple 30-minute workout, then I'm going to do one push-up. Great job, Stephen. You can do a push-up. Your dreams will surely come true now.

As I lowered myself to the ground, my joints creaked, my arms were weak, and my body screamed at me to sit on the couch… but all I had to do was one push-up. So I did, and it transformed my life.

While in push-up position, it seemed silly to do a single push-up, so I did a few more, then stood up. At this point, I was intrigued. This was the same way I would have started a 30-minute workout. I had already met and exceeded my goal, and my body was warmed up. I set a few more small goals and my push-up count reached 50 reps. After that, I grabbed my pull-up bar and did the same thing. A full 20 minutes of exercise later, I faced the ultimate challenge.

I had the idea to do a 10-minute ab program to finish off my workout, but my brain shot it down like a professional skeet shooter. *You've had your fun with exercise, Stephen, but I'm drawing the line here. Go play video games.*

Resistance was strong, but I'm a quick learner. I used my new secret weapon, and made sure to compliment my subconscious (the source of resistance). My thought process went something like this.

1. *Oh mighty subconscious, I wouldn't dare exercise my abs for 10 minutes, but would you mind if I just set up my exercise mat?*
2. *Oh great brain of legend, now that my mat is set up, would it be alright to sit on it?*
3. *Oh tremendous cranial overlord, is there any harm in finding an ab exercise video on YouTube and pressing Play?*

Bingo. It worked. 10 minutes later, my abdominal muscles were ablaze. I sat on my bed with a glass of water and took it in: **My one push-up had somehow grown into the 30-minute workout that I was unable to do before.** My brain nearly exploded out of surprise and delight. I had broken through an amount of resistance that I had *never* overcome previously. That situation had always meant failure, but this time, I succeeded. What could this mean for my future?

From that day on, I vowed to do at least one push-up every day. Admittedly, I missed two days in the next six months, but otherwise, I always did my push-up(s). Sometimes, it would spark a full workout as it did the first time. Other times, I would only do five to 10. On a few occasions, I did just one push-up to meet my requirement.

A Pleasant Surprise

I was already happy about one measly push-up sparking full workouts and more exercise; then I noticed something even more exciting. The baseline level of resistance I felt to exercise had decreased significantly over time. When considering exercise, I no longer felt repulsed. How could I? It was now part of my life and I did it in varying amounts every day. I knew I was ready for the next step.

After roughly six months of doing one push-up per day, I began going to the gym. To this day, unless I'm traveling, sick, or injured, I go to the gym several times per week. My unwillingness to exercise is no longer an obstacle.

When one push-up morphed into a full gym habit, my already-wide eyes grew to the size of bowling balls (you should see the picture). Just as I had leveraged small steps into a big change, I knew I could leverage this *entire concept* to improve different areas of my life. I immediately began daily goals of reading two pages in a book per day and writing 50 words per day. My reading and writing activity spiked. As a long-time writer, I had been thinking for the previous year about writing a personal development book, but couldn't decide on a topic. Well, I certainly had one now!

Using my 50 words per day goal, I wrote a book about this concept called *Mini Habits: Smaller Habits, Bigger Results*. That's right: I used a mini habit to write *Mini Habits*. The words poured out of my soul. I was excited to tell others about this discovery, and scared that nobody would read it or believe it.

Since it was a ridiculous premise, but I knew it worked, I researched habit formation, willpower, and motivation, and it all came together. This crazy "one push-up a day" idea actually had scientific merit! This made me even more excited to share it because if I could explain exactly *how* it worked, people might believe my story, try it themselves, and change their lives. The book was published on December 22, 2013, almost exactly a year after I did that single push-up that changed my life.

Luckily, a lot of people did read it. *Mini Habits* has become a worldwide bestseller, selling more than 125,000 copies in its first two years in over a dozen languages and becoming the #1 selling self-help book in three countries. This was my first book, and its success is a reflection of the success readers have had with it. People changed their lives with this strategy, and shared it with others.

The mini habits strategy is different from 99.9% of self-help content because it emphasizes consistency over *all else*. Other books that correctly promote consistency don't usually have a thoughtful application strategy for it. Importantly, *Mini Habits* doesn't merely say "be consistent"—it is woven into the fabric of the strategy.

What does any of this have to do with weight loss? More than even I thought when I started writing this book. It turns out that behavior change and biological change work in much the same way, and the strategic mistakes that prevent people from changing their behavior also prevent them from losing weight. For example, when people forcibly restrict their calories, they almost always gain the weight back, just as someone reverts to their typical way of living after trying to force themselves to reach ambitious goals.

Why Lose Weight?

Being overweight is not a crime. It doesn't lower your value as a human being. Weight, however, *can* affect your health. It *can* affect your ability to do and/or enjoy activities. It *can* affect your self-esteem. It *can* affect nearly all aspects of your life.

If you want to lose weight, do it for yourself. Don't do it because you're "supposed to be thinner" or have a certain body mass index (BMI). There is no rule that states "Thou shalt have a BMI between 18.5 and 25." Body weight is a shallow, incomplete measure of a person's health. Some exceptionally muscular and fit people are actually considered overweight or even obese according to their BMI.

When you say you want to lose weight, what you really mean is that you want to play with your kids without getting winded, you want to look in the mirror and feel good about what you see, you want to impress someone, you want to live a long and healthy life, you want to improve your overall quality of life, or you want to look good in spandex. These are all fine reasons to lose weight as long as they come from you.

Book Structure

There are two parts to this book. Part one covers weight loss: current popular methods, why they're broken, how the brain and body naturally change, how weight loss works, and the resulting best approach.

Part two covers strategies that are based on the conclusions of part one. We'll begin part two with the ideal psychology of weight loss. How should we think about our weight loss journey in general? How should we approach food and fitness? Once these questions are thoroughly gone into, you'll have a solid idea of not only the best way to lose weight, but the best mindset for weight loss. For example, you'll know that processed food is a major cause of weight gain, but also that you shouldn't try to resist it directly.

At this point, you'll be ready to formulate your mini habits plan, and there's an in-depth guide to help you create a plan that suits your lifestyle. Unlike dieting, a mini habit plan is completely flexible and adaptable *to you*. Once you've got a mini habit plan, we'll talk about situational strategies, like how to handle holidays, snacking, temptation, peer pressure, eating out, and buying groceries.

Some books give you recipes. Some books give you a list of foods to (not) eat. This book teaches you how to change your behavior to lose weight permanently, and that's more valuable than the world's greatest recipe book or most accurate list of weight loss foods. When you can change your behavior, you can become the person you've always wanted to become.

The techniques in this book are powerful and transformative, and yet they're so simple that anyone can succeed with them.

Part One

Introduction: Diet's Two Definitions

Before we begin, to avoid confusion, we need to define the two ways people use the word "diet."

1. Diet (n): food and drink regularly provided or consumed
2. Diet (v): to eat less food or to eat only particular kinds of food in order to lose weight[1]

Every single person has a diet (#1), but not everyone is on a diet (#2). The second definition is also known as "dieting." The easiest way to think of it is that #1 is a noun and #2 is a verb. Dieting or "going on a diet" is something you may or may not do, but a diet is a noun that every person possesses.

I mention this so you don't think I'm contradicting myself as I verbally destroy the practice of "dieting" (v) and then suggest a particular type of diet (n) for weight loss. To "go on a diet" or start "dieting" means that you're consciously modifying your food type or amount. It's one specific (and ineffective) strategy to change your diet (n) and lose weight. **If you determine a particular diet is ideal for weight loss, dieting is NOT the only way to get yourself to eat that way.**

Mini Habits for Weight Loss is not training wheels for those who can't stick to a diet; this is the advanced program. It's entirely different and much smarter than dieting, with a higher success rate. Dieting is for temporary weight loss. We're aiming for real, lasting change.

1

The Unhappy Marriage of Weight Loss and Dieting

Dieting and Smoothie Cleanses Are Effective for Weight Gain. Wait... What?

"It isn't that they can't see the solution. It is that they can't see the problem."
~ Gilbert K. Chesterton

Dieting Makes Us Fat

Brace yourself, because this will shock you.

In 1986, scientists sought to find the metabolic impact of yo-yo dieting. To simulate this behavior, which is marked by repeated weight loss and regain, they alternately restricted and expanded the calorie consumption of obese rats. The rats completed two full "yo-yo" weight loss cycles.

To lose weight the first time, rats were fed 50% of the average food consumption of control rats until they had lost 131 grams of weight. Once the rats regained that weight, they used the same 50% restriction for the second weight loss cycle, and the rats lost 133 grams. That's almost the same, right? Yes, but the amount of weight gained or lost—the typical focus of dieters—was not the focal point here. Instead, the scientists looked at *how long* it took the rats to lose weight in each cycle (using the same diet). They wanted to see how yo-yo dieting affected the rats' metabolism, if it changed the rats' *propensity* to lose (or gain) weight. It changed significantly, and not for the better.

It took the rats 21 days to lose 131g the first time. The second time—which used the same exact calorie restriction diet—took 46 days, more than twice as long. The effect was even worse for the weight gain part of the cycle. After the first weight loss, the rats took 29 days to regain their pre-diet weight. After their second weight loss, it only took them 10 days to regain the weight.

By losing and regaining weight repeatedly, the rats' bodies became more than twice as resistant to weight loss and almost three times as prone to weight gain (by function of time on identical diets).[2]

Cycling weight gain and loss increased the rats' food efficiency, meaning that the rats' bodies became more conservative with the energy they took in and stored as much fat as ratly possible. This is the opposite goal of a person (or rat) trying to lose weight, but it's the natural biological response of a starved or partially starved animal. If you lived in a time when famines were common, such increased food efficiency could save your life. But for those of us who have an abundance of food and artificially restrict our intake to lose weight, well, that *still* tells our metabolism to slow down and not burn too many calories because, for all it knows, the next meal might not be coming anytime soon.

This study is one of many to find weight-gaining metabolic shifts in rats from calorie restriction yo-yoing. [3]Thankfully, this is just rats and has nothing to do with humans, or else someone would have told us 30 years ago, right? Wrong. This biological mechanism affects us, too.

Every person should know about this analysis, but few do. Consider this: UCLA researchers looked at *31 long-term studies* on dieting and found that, across the studies, dieting caused 33% to 66% of participants to regain more weight than they lost while dieting.[4] If those numbers seem bad, well, they're almost certainly *worse* than that. Many of the participants they followed up with were contacted years after their study's conclusion. Not all participants reported back about their weight change, and who do you think would be least likely to report back? The ashamed ones who regained the most weight.

"These studies likely underestimate the extent to which dieting is counterproductive because of several methodological problems, all of which bias the studies toward showing successful weight loss maintenance."

A three-year study of almost 15,000 children aged 9-14 found that those who dieted were more prone to binge eating.[5] Those who dieted, male and female, frequent and infrequent, gained more weight across the board in the study's duration. That is strike two against dieting (or are we at four yet?).

Another study compared twins, which is interesting, because it takes genetics out of the equation. Over 4,000 individual Finnish twins were monitored for 25 years. The twin halves who attempted intentional weight loss (dieting) gained more weight than their genetically identical siblings, and weight gain increased with subsequent dieting attempts.[6] The dieting halves probably increased their desire for foods that would make them gain weight by depriving themselves of them.

In a 1944 study called the Minnesota Starvation Experiment, 36 male volunteers were semi-starved for 24 weeks. One of the primary observations was that most of the men became depressed and emotionally distressed.[7] At least they lost weight, right? Right! Predictably, yes and then no.

For 24 weeks, the men ate only 1,600 calories per day (which isn't enough for grown men). They did lose a lot of weight at first, but then their bodies responded as bodies always do to sustained calorie restriction: "The men lost an average of a pound of body fat a week over the first 12 weeks, but averaged only a quarter-pound per week over the next 12, despite the continued deprivation."[8] When the men's bodies increased their food efficiency (remember the rats?), their rate of weight loss slowed to a crawl. (Those watching their waistline see this as a bad thing, but it's actually a phenomenal survival adaptation.)

At the conclusion of the study, the men were allowed to recover and eat to satiety, and they ate up to 10,000 calories a day. What else does that tell you about their bodies' response? If their bodies could speak throughout this experiment, they'd say, "Famine! Conserve as much energy as possible, and when you have access to food, gorge on it and store it as fat in case the famine persists!" That's exactly what happened. They bounced back to their former weight rapidly, and then some. They accumulated 50% more body fat than they had before the study began. Yikes!

The Biggest Loser is a hit American TV show with millions of viewers. It has been one of the most successful reality TV shows of all time. The premise: Which contestant can lose the most weight by show's end?

What do you think is the recipe for weight loss on the show, the one that produces massive double-digit and even triple-digit weight loss numbers in a short amount of time? It's the same one we just covered. Exercise for hours every day and severely restrict your calorie intake to create a big calorie deficit.[9] Yep, that will do it! Considering the information we've just covered, go ahead and take a guess about what happens to these contestants during and after the show.

During the show, contestants lose a massive amount of weight, some of them dropping well over 100 pounds. What happens next?

A study followed 14 *Biggest Loser* contestants for six years after the show, and all but one of them regained weight after the show.[10] Four became *heavier* than when they started the show. Even worse, nearly all of them suffered from abnormally low metabolism for their size, and lower metabolism than when they started. Low metabolism makes weight loss much, much harder, and weight gain effortless.

When this study came out in May 2016, I saw *Good Morning America* discuss it, and those on the show acted as if we hadn't known about this concept for decades. My first thought was, "Why are they acting surprised?"

Thirty years ago, we saw this exact same thing happen with rats. Forty years before *that*, we saw it happen in the Minnesota Starvation Experiment (1944). We *already knew* that when you semi-starve an animal, its body reacts by slowing metabolism, increasing hunger, and storing as much fat energy as possible to increase its odds of survival. This isn't *merely* common sense—and it is that—it's also proven science.

Even worse, we've generated a pessimistic view that all weight loss attempts are futile because people will regain the weight later. But that's because our notion of how to lose weight is too narrow. It's like saying that every time you start a fire, it will become a forest fire (because you only start fires in the middle of dry forests). If you do something wrong, you'll get terrible results every time.

If you want to get fatter, try dieting. Buy the books that promise "X pounds lost in X days." The science clearly supports these methods for weight gain. What's that? You want weight *loss*? Oh. To do that, you'll need a different strategy.

Imagine that you were one of the rats in the yo-yo dieting study. If you had just seen firsthand what diet cycling did to you, and someone told you about a semi-starvation smoothie "cleanse" that could help you lose 15 pounds in 10 days, what would your reaction be?

Imagine that you were one of the men in the Minnesota Starvation Experiment. Would you adopt a calorie-restriction diet to lose the fat you gained from… having a calorie-restriction diet? Didn't Albert Einstein once say something profound about doing the same thing repeatedly and expecting a different result? Their suffering aside, it must have been shocking to gain so much fat so fast after semi-starving themselves for months! Maybe you have already experienced this same unfortunate weight gain effect from diet cycling, but you probably attributed your weight struggles to other things because you assumed dieting was the only way.

Let this soak in. Anyone who says they're going on a diet has a great chance of *gaining weight* because of it. This is not an opinion. This is what the data shows. The true cost of following short-term weight loss solutions isn't merely wasted time, effort, and momentary suffering, it's all that plus further weight gain. The people and rats in these studies had *the dream scenario* for dieting—they had their calories controlled for them, so they wouldn't have to fight themselves to eat less, and all it did was make them fatter in the end. All of them. And calorie restriction, ladies and gentlemen, is the most common strategy for weight loss worldwide. Sigh.

Calorie restriction isn't the main problem, it's just one part of the bigger "dieting" problem. There are some quality, nutritious diets out there with the potential to bring lasting weight loss. But if so many people are on wholesome, nutrition-based diets, why do obesity rates continue to rise?

Simple. The crux of weight loss is not whether or not you eat blueberries or grapes. It's not about if you're a slow carb, low carb, low calorie, paleo, or Mediterranean diet aficionado. It's not about if you can eat the perfect diet for 30 days. The crux of weight loss is whether or not you can sustain healthy lifestyle changes in the long term. Go about it the wrong way, and not only will you lose time, but you'll also screw up your metabolism or your view of healthy food in the process. (If you've already done that, you can reverse this damage with the right strategy. The body and mind are capable self-healers.)

Let's get to the root of the problem, then.

Why Dieting Is Broken

If you look for weight loss books, what will you find?

*   "The BLAH Diet"
*   "The NEW BLAH BLAH Diet"
*   "We Decided That This Diet Will Last 30 Days Because... Reasons!"
*   "Celebrity Diet #283: Buy it Because She's Famous!"

The marketplace is saturated with **dieting** books. Amazon's category name is even called "Weight Loss & Dieting," as if weight loss has fallen in love with dieting, they're getting married, and any other suitors are too late.

Are there any who object to this union? I do. Vehemently so!

The marriage of weight loss and dieting is sad, because the entire concept of dieting is broken. As with some spouses, it doesn't work. At the risk of giving relationship advice in a weight loss book, healthy couples make each other *better*. The dieting industry makes billions of dollars every year, despite being ineffective. How many people believe it's impossible to lose weight and keep it off because dieting failed them? There are a lot of frustrated people because of this failed marriage.

Does Dieting Ever Work Long-Term?

Since many scientists assume dieting is "the way," short-term studies are used to try to validate its various forms. A. Janet Tomiyama reports in *American Psychologist*: "Several studies that are often cited as support for the long-term success of diets followed individuals for less than one year, six months, or even less time."[11]

There's an overabundance of short-term studies on weight loss and dieting, because we don't like the results of long-term studies. A 7.5-year study found that women who had consumed a low-fat diet weighed only one pound less than those on a typical Western diet.[12] Studies on dieting have found that most diets work well in the short term, whether they're based on calorie restriction or eating better foods. But they generally don't work long-term, because they're so poorly designed.

We're in this situation because of a chronic short-term focus. Even on a consumer and personal level, people are making major life decisions based upon seeing a friend drop 12 pounds in two weeks on a smoothie cleanse. Oy vey, people!

Do you know the **single most effective** short-term weight loss solution? Don't eat any food and work out for two hours a day. You will lose more weight faster than you've ever lost it before in your life! With my new diet, The Newest New No-Food-Necessary Diet™, you'll lose weight so quickly it's dangerous (literally). Lose up to 20 pounds in one week! It really works! I hope my sarcasm is clear. Do NOT try The Newest New No-Food-Necessary Diet™. Some people would scoff at this idea as if it's absurd, when they're doing *this exact thing* to a lesser degree (e.g., calorie-restriction diets or masked calorie-restriction diets such as cleanses).

Short-term solutions are as worthless for weight loss as our fence was for keeping our family dog, Shiloh "Houdini" Guise, in our backyard (she'd jump over our 6-foot fence and swim around in the local lake). Just because a diet says 30 days instead of a week or lets you drink a few green smoothies instead of completely starving yourself, that doesn't make it any more sustainable. Weight loss plans are either sustainable for you or they aren't—it's black and white—and almost every weight loss plan out there is unsustainable, superficial, and a waste of your time.

The Wrong Focal Point

Have you noticed that the only two variables the weight loss industry is bent on changing are the type or quantity of food we consume? Book after book after book tells you it's the carbs, it's the meat, it's the calories, it's the wheat! Here's the formula.

1. A new dieting book comes out.
2. The book explains why other diets don't work—too many carbs, not enough fish oil, too much fruit, too little fruit, the wrong ratio of macronutrients, insufficient diet soda intake, too many calories, not enough exercise, too much wheat, etc.
3. The book presents a new theory about the "ideal diet."

Nothing is inherently wrong with this process. It makes sense to question the foods we eat and seek the ideal ones for our health and weight. This, however, is the wrong focal point. *We don't need the perfect diet formula; we need an alternative to the broken dieting method.* Even those books with clever titles about being the "non-diet solution" to weight loss proceed to incorporate the exact same *principles of dieting* into their "non-diet." Most commonly, they'll give you a list of foods to eat and not eat and some sort of unsustainable application plan (with a cheat day if you're lucky).

We've mistaken the diet (n) as the problem to be solved, which has introduced way too much complexity into what has always been a simple truth (eat real, whole foods to lose weight). We have hundreds of diets (n) —many of which recognize the basic correct foods to eat—but they share the same broken dieting (v) strategies.

The broken concept of dieting is to attempt to quickly switch from one way of eating to another, often (but not always) for a set period of time.

Whether it's a plan designed for life or one for 10-30 days, it's usually: *Eat this way and you'll lose weight. Get motivated. Do it. Good luck!*

This is a lousy strategy that consistently fails, and people have tried everything to get it to work.

Some make diet plans in which there are no rules and you just try to eat the right foods. This is closer to a real solution because it's flexible, but it isn't structured or strategic enough to change behavior.

Others try to take your decision-making out of the process. This can work for some time, but eventually, people will make their own food choices. Taking away your freedom to choose is rarely effective, because you can take back your power of choice at any time. It's better to change the way you make decisions.

Some ignore the *types* of foods we eat and simplify the goal to counting calories, but calorie counting is a pain to maintain, it's inaccurate, it doesn't focus on proper nutrition, and, as we just covered, it causes long-term weight gain. In his book *The Calorie Myth*, Jonathan Bailor succinctly describes the accuracy problem with calorie counting: "Since the late 1970s, we have gradually worked our way up to eating an additional 570 calories per day. But let's estimate that over those few decades, we each ate a more modest 300 additional calories per day. According to traditional calorie math, the average American should have gained 907 pounds of fat between 1977 and 2006."[13] That didn't happen because traditional calorie math is bunk. Our bodies are not calculators. It's not "calories in, calories out" (CICO); it's more like "calories in, complex biological reactions, calories out."

If you've quit dieting, you've probably told yourself that it was too strict, too complicated, or too bland. That is probably true, but the flawed assumption underlying those thoughts is that you'll *ever* find "the right diet." Let me just tell you: The next popular dieting book won't work any better than the previous ones, because it won't focus on sustainability.

The best weight loss books will tell you—as creatively as possible and with just enough twists to make them seem "unique"—that processed foods make us sicker and fatter, while whole foods help create leaner, healthier bodies. Such a change in diet (n) is necessary for results, but, like with every other change, it's the strategy of implementation that makes or breaks weight loss plans. To succeed, we must gently reroute the habitual eating patterns that cause weight gain.

These Meta-Analyses Say It All

A meta-analysis is a "study of studies." Meta-analyses are some of the most useful and reliable pieces of scientific data. It seems that any single study can validate or invalidate almost any point of view, and the data from different studies can be contradictory, but if something holds true over almost every study in that field, then there's a very good chance it's a correct and true observation.

There have been some meta-analyses done on weight loss diets. They looked at different diets to find the most effective one, but there was a problem that made the "best diet" question a moot point. **Both analyses found that people don't stick with their diets long-term.**

One said, "Almost half of the studies included in our meta-analysis had completion rates less than 70%."[14] You might think that less than 70% isn't too bad, but it is actually *awful* when you consider that these are short-term *studies*. People were being counted on to provide data and insight into a big problem. They had extra accountability and motivation to stick to their diet, they only had to do it for a limited time, and they *still* dropped out. If so many people are failing in that scenario, how much harder is it for the person trying to change on their own with little external motivation and support?

In a commentary on another meta-analysis done on 53 studies involving 68,128 adults, Dr. Kevin Hall concluded, "What seems to be clear is that long-term diet adherence is abysmal, irrespective of whether low-fat or other diets, such as low-carbohydrate diets, are prescribed."[15] Even when people correctly avoid yo-yoing their calorie intake, they can't seem to consistently eat well on nutrition-based diets. They're failing to change their behavior.

Why do we trust the framework that's been failing us for decades as obesity continues to march on unchallenged? We've got the wrong guy! The diet formulas are constantly blamed and pitted against one another. Low-carb camps say low-fat dieting doesn't work, and low-fat camps say Paleo is ineffective, while Paleo screams at low-calorie diets as the problem. We're blaming the ball for passing through a shredded racket. Let's first get a racket that can hit things, and then maybe we can worry about the ball.

The failure of the weight loss industry is not the fault of diets (n), it's the fault of *dieting* (v). Many of these diets will work well if you stick to them, but you can't just "do whatever it takes" to stick to them. We need a smarter application strategy that infiltrates our underlying habitual and biological systems like a ninja. That's where we run into another problem: Conventional habit formation advice is also ineffective (we'll discuss why in chapter two), so even if it were properly integrated into weight loss solutions (it's not), it wouldn't work well.

Where Do We Go from Here?

Is the lesson here not to attempt to lose weight? If you're going to be dieting, then yes, you're better off not doing that. If you've tried one diet, you've basically tried them all. But *Mini Habits for Weight Loss* is not a dieting book, so the discouraging data on dieting doesn't apply to it. There is very little research on the impact of small, consistent, lasting changes for weight loss, because it's not dieting. I did find a couple of promising ones, though.

One small study followed three groups, and the group implementing small changes lost significantly more weight than the control group and the traditional dieting group, but the follow-up was only three months. Their changes were sustained at three months, but following up for a longer time would have been helpful.[16]

A little-known but enlightening study showed a linear relationship between consistency in diet and successful weight loss and maintenance.[17] Researchers looked at the National Weight Control Registry of people with successful long-term weight loss and found that "participants who reported a consistent diet across the week were 1.5 times more likely to maintain their weight within 5 pounds over the subsequent year than participants who dieted more strictly on weekdays."

Consistency is not only the key to behavior change: it is evidence of behavior change. Those trying to force themselves to eat a certain way will often slip up and have "cheat days," when they eat what they want to eat. Those who succeed change their underlying food preferences through the power of habit formation.

It's time for a new approach. It's time for *Mini Habits*. We're going to apply the world's most effective change strategy to one of the world's biggest problems. This is the marriage we've needed all along. It is a fundamentally different approach to weight loss, not in its recommendation of what foods to eat (though I will discuss it), but in its strategy for changing your dietary and movement habits.

Since this will almost certainly be the only book I write on weight loss, I have no incentive to trick you with short-term success. There are no plans to follow up this book with *Xtreme Smoothie Fat Blasting Slim Belly Ripper Detox Cleanse 2.0: Become Completely Weightless in Just 14 Days!* (unless I take up writing parodies). My incentive is to give you a timeless solution that lasts a lifetime and enables you to change your body and brain at a natural pace.

The Mini Habits Connection to Weight Loss

Successful weight loss requires a new set of habits. Your current and past habits have created your current weight. A different set of habits will create a different result (ideally, some rate of weight loss).

Mini habits will help you build a powerful new habitual base for healthy living. I'm not going to guarantee you won't gain weight back once you change with mini habits, because **no person is immune to gaining weight at any time**. Closely tied to that, no person is beyond reverting back to old habits, because unhealthy food still tastes pretty good, even after you develop your healthy spinach addiction. Weight loss strategies are like fortresses: none is *invincible* to setbacks and problems, but the mini habits fortress is strong, reliable, and resilient.

The One Requirement for Lasting Change
Lasting change requires only one thing: consistent action over time. A mini habit is designed to fit this requirement exactly, making it the simplest, easiest, and overall ultimate vehicle for behavior change. To show you its power, these are my real life results with mini habits (as of writing, all of them are still in effect more than two years after starting).

- I've had a consistent gym habit for more than two years and I'm in the best shape of my life.
- I've written two international bestselling books and hundreds of blog posts. I've written a new blog post every week for two years straight without missing a week.
- I read 12-20 books a year now, after typically reading only one per year.

That's what I got, which is exceptional relative to my past, and this is the laughable way I got it.

- Fitness mini habit: one push-up per day
- Writing mini habit: 50 words per day
- Reading mini habit: two pages per day

The most significant accomplishments of my life were achieved with three behaviors that require a cumulative time of *less than five minutes to accomplish each day*. These are mini habits. People have gotten even better results than I have with their mini habits, which doesn't seem fair since I wrote the book. Kidding aside, I'm ecstatic to hear the success stories. Some people didn't even wait for this book to come out before figuring out how to use mini habits to lose weight. Bravo!

How is it possible for something so small to become so significant? Compounding.

The Sneaky Power of Compounding
Imagine you have a choice between getting the sum of one penny that's doubled for 31 days or a lump sum of $5 million. Shockingly, you'd be crazy to take the $5 million, because in 31 days, your penny will have doubled its way to over $10 million. (Hat tip to Darren Hardy's *The Compound Effect* for the example.) This intriguing fact reveals the problem and the solution for all of life.

The solution for life is to focus on compounding small choices in the direction desired. The problem is that we don't see this solution, because we are easily impressed with the highly visible things like $5 million, and naturally less intrigued by the (counterintuitively) more powerful small and compoundable changes.

Think about this in terms of gaining a pound every month versus losing a pound every month. After one year, you'd weigh 12 pounds more or less. And the difference between these two scenarios is *24 pounds*. That's a significant difference for a small change in weight from one month to the next; our weight can fluctuate more than one pound in a single day!

One pound gained or lost only represents linear growth. Because of momentum, emotions, and accrued experience, forward progress is often *exponential*. It will compound. To put it into real terms, how do you think it would feel to be 12 pounds lighter than you are right now? How would it impact the way you feel about yourself? How do you think it would affect your energy levels? How do you think it would change your motivation and willingness to go further? Depending on which direction you go, just one pound gained or lost per month will put you well ahead or well behind, physically and psychologically, after one year.

Your food and exercise decisions can create a greater difference than one pound gained or lost per month. **The fact that one pound per month is enough to create such a massive difference means that every meal decision matters.** The smallest choices make the biggest difference.

Don't misinterpret this. Aiming for one pound lost a month is not the suggestion here. For one, it's too vague a focus. Compounded results are great, but they must start somewhere specific. If you double a penny every day for 31 days, you get more than $10 million. If you double nothing for 31 days, you get *nothing*. That little penny isn't just important, *it's everything*.

Permanent Improvement
If you succeed with *Mini Habits for Weight Loss*, it will become a matter of simply living out your new identity, which automatically and naturally produces a healthier version of you.

This internal change is more important than fat loss. Wise people recognize that who we are matters more than what we look like. Nobody escapes the detrimental effects of aging, so if all you care about is looking good, time is already going to ruin your plan. I'm not saying you shouldn't pursue the healthy body of your dreams—do it—I'm just saying that the outside-in approach is destined for failure.

The person who loses weight by superficial ploys like diet pills, surgery, or starvation may feel excited at early results, but they won't feel overwhelmed with joy about *how* they got those results, and they'll feel terrible when they inevitably regain the weight. When you orchestrate a real and lasting improvement in your life, you'll be surprised that the outer change actually takes a back seat to the joy of inner growth, which alters *who we are*. Inner growth affects *our identity*. You may not believe me now, but that will ultimately matter more to you than what the scale ever said.

We'll discuss how change works in the next chapter. It's important to establish our philosophy of behavior change before we even get to weight loss and how that works. It doesn't matter what your plan is if you can't change your behavior, so let's nail that down first.

2
Brain Change before Body Change

Get Motivated? Get Out of Here!

"Habit is stronger than reason."
~ Georga Santayana

How Change Doesn't Work

In this book, you won't find...

- Exclusive recipes
- Calorie counting plans
- "The One" Diet to Rule Them All
- Demonization of carbs or fat as the single culprit of all obesity

The big "ah-ha!" factor of this book is one that other weight loss books lack: you're going to get actionable strategies that mesh with your current lifestyle to help you achieve *lasting* change. I will cover the nutrition and weight impact of some foods, but if you firmly believe that a particular diet (n) is the best one for you, feel free to combine it with the strategies found in this book instead of "going on a diet." (Ditch their suggested implementation plan and create a mini habit plan instead.) Beyond knowing the basic mechanisms behind weight gain and loss, losing weight comes down to whether or not you can permanently change your behavior.

Results in 30 Days or Less?

If you see "X pounds in X days" on a book, burn it immediately (or sneer at it if it's digital). For the love of kale, *please* don't ever aim for 7, 10, 21, or 30 days of change! The best use of a 30-day plan is if you have 30 days left to live. In the context of a life of about 28,000 days, 30 days' worth of change is exactly as worthless as it looks.

I understand the theory that people will act differently for 30 days, and after that, they'll have formed a habit or be motivated enough to keep the changes. But there is no scientific evidence that habits are formed in 30 or 21 days.[18] A 2009 study found that participants took an average of 66 days to form a habit, with a wild range of 18 to 254 days.[19] That tells us two things: the brain changes fairly slowly, but the exact speed at which it does for any given behavior is unpredictable. There's a great chance a new behavior *won't* be habitual by day 30.

Also, people like to make 30-day challenges difficult, since they only have to do it for a limited time. This makes habit formation even more unlikely. The above study found that the speed of habit formation is greatly influenced by the difficulty of the behavior. The brain will be much faster to adopt an easy habit of drinking one glass of water every morning (about 20 days according to the study) than to develop the challenging habit of practicing upside-down Kung Fu for two hours every day after dinner.

Legendary Chinese war general Sun Tzu once said, "Victorious warriors win first and then go to war, while defeated warriors go to war first and then seek to win." Change is not about being able to fight yourself for 30 days; it's about getting so strategic that you win before the fight begins. **Applied to us, the key to losing weight is to change your brain before trying to change your body.**

The Brain Change Process

If your body is the result of your brain state, how does the brain change?

Your subconscious brain is the boss, because it directly drives about half of your behavior and is constantly influencing your conscious decisions. People always try to fight against it, and they lose. Our strategy is to change it using its own nature, not cultural ideas like, "You just gotta want it more, bro!"

What is the true nature of the brain? The brain is a slow-changing machine, and that's a good thing. If your brain could completely change overnight, *you would be unstable.* Let's just say that your norm is to wake up, read the paper with coffee and a bagel, walk your dog, and watch the news. This is your habitual routine. Then one night, you get a phone call at 3 AM and have to run outside in your underwear to check on your neighbors. What if your brain latched on to this new routine and you continued to run outside at 3 AM every night in your underwear? Nobody would want that, so it's a good thing our brains require more repetition than that! Let's accept and be thankful for the stability our slow-changing brains provide us.

The ideal brain change process is so gradual that you may not notice it! This is a *good* thing. The more noticeable a change—such as when you switch from burgers and fries to "only green juice"—the more your brain is going to try to shut it down. (Just to clarify, it's fine to juice vegetables as additional nutrition to a regular diet. There may even be health benefits in juice fasting for a day or two, but it is absolutely not a sustainable weight loss solution.)

The Tyranny of Motivation

I'm going to let you in on a dark secret of humanity—or perhaps you already know it. Most people are terrible... let me finish... at reaching their goals. For example, New Year's Resolutions have a reported 92% failure rate.[20]

Change attempts fail frequently, and when they do, others tend to assume it's because the person was lazy or not motivated enough to follow through with the change. But most plans fail because they aren't designed to fit the brain's change process. It's like saying, "Here's a plan to stop bullets—simply catch them in your teeth!" (It will only work if you're Superman.) **The value of a solution is dependent on its implementability. The "greatest idea" is actually worthless if it can't be executed (teleportation, for example).**

Brain change must precede body change or the changes won't last. Since the brain is changed by consistent action over time, the question is: How does one take action consistently? We can deduce the answer.

Willpower and motivation are the two mechanisms by which we consciously take action (i.e., actions not from habit). Motivation is the *desire* to act (our default choice). Willpower is the *decision* to act regardless of feelings. Nearly every self-help book in existence (weight loss books included) suggests generating as much motivation as possible and using willpower as a backup plan. It's a bad idea to rely on motivation first.

The Undeserved Popularity of "Getting Motivated"
I bet you've heard of motivational speakers. Out of curiosity, how many discipline or willpower speakers have you heard of? The number of motivational books, websites, and podcasts dwarf any other self-help topic (except perhaps weight loss).[21]

Let me make one thing clear: The popularity of motivation is because of its perceived track record, not its actual one. For every motivational success story you read, there are many more failure stories. If a strategy has a 2% success rate, but the 98% are ignored, our perspective of that strategy's effectiveness will be (and has been) extremely distorted. The failures don't have stories written about them, but here's one for you: I

28

made very little progress in 10 years trying to "get motivated."

Deceptive success rates don't only happen on a person-by-person basis. People experience the same phenomenon on a micro level in their own lives. **It's on the days you feel motivated and then pursue your goals that you take notice and think, "Motivation is the key to action!"**

It's natural to pay attention to what works, so when you eat a healthy meal after feeling motivated to reach your weight loss goals, you'll attribute the behavior (eating healthy food) to the motivation you felt just before it. It only makes sense to emulate what's been successful in the past, right? Yes, but only if you consider the entirety of the data (not just one data point).

It's dangerous to draw conclusions from individual events. For example, if you bet $5 on the number 20 in roulette and the ball settles into the 20 slot, you'll win $175. But are you going to conclude that the ball always lands on 20? Are you going to conclude that the ball lands on 20 more often than on the other numbers? Do that and you'll go broke in Vegas. In the same way, if you happen to "get motivated" one morning out of 20 mornings, or even 10 mornings out of 20 mornings, why would you assume the strategy is successful? It may be because you don't know any other way, or because you put too much faith in your ability to "get motivated" at will.

Just to be clear, I am not anti-motivational. I feel motivated as I write this! Motivation is a wholly good thing that benefits us. I am simply calling it out as a poor basis for behavior change. Foundations must be reliable, and motivation is not reliable. That's all. Why, then, do we think that motivation is reliable?

Familiarity, The Great Deceiver

Pulitzer Prize winner Daniel Kahneman says in *Thinking, Fast and Slow*, "A reliable way to make people believe in falsehoods is frequent repetition, because familiarity is not easily distinguished from truth."[22] Once a concept's popularity ascends to a certain point, people will blindly assume its truth, and no amount of valid criticism can fully eradicate it. Such is the case with getting motivated as a behavior change strategy. (Everyone used to think Earth is flat, but that one was simpler to disprove.)

Motivated people who succeed tend to confuse the symptom for the cause and say, "My desire fueled me." The truth? Success and good habits fuel desire far more often than the reverse.

Do We Want it Enough?

Mainstream motivational theory states that, in order to enact change, one must simply "want it more." If you fail to reach a goal, it's your fault for not wanting it enough. As the world is suffering from obesity and its related diseases, we must not want to change enough. It's a pity that we're not motivated enough to save our own lives and live better. But wait… the weight loss industry made $64 billion in 2014.[23] When that much money is spent on something, it means public interest is through the thermosphere.

Sadly, in this very moment, millions if not billions of people are wondering what's wrong with them. Nothing is wrong with them! These people have *willingly suffered and paid money* trying to lose weight, and they are *still* being told their desire for change isn't strong enough![24] That's so wrong it's criminal. People have plenty of desire; they just need a smart strategy that doesn't rely on doing the impossible.

To fully understand motivation, we need to distinguish its two different types.

The Two Types of Motivation

Look at this sentence: I'm motivated to *quit smoking*, and I'm motivated to *smoke this cigarette right now*.

These are not merely contradicting motivations; they are different *types* of motivation. Motivation to quit smoking is a *general desire*. Motivation to smoke a cigarette is a *momentary desire*.

Momentary motivation is far more complex than general motivation. Your in-the-moment desire to do or not do something will be influenced by *multiple* contextual and general desires. For example, your choice to eat a doughnut right now could be influenced by your motivation to…

- Be healthy: you don't want to eat it!
- Eat something tasty: you want to eat it!
- Feel good: you want to eat it!
- Fit in with your friends who are eating doughnuts: you want to eat it!

- Avoid weight gain: you don't want to eat it!
- Get ready for beach season: you don't want to eat it!

Other factors include your stress level, internal dialogue, and emotional state. Consider your experience: What happens to your motivation to do positive things when you're having a bad day? It decreases. On a good day, it increases. And have you experienced random motivation drops for seemingly no reason? Me too. It's because emotion drives much of the momentary motivation equation. Momentary motivation is messy, complex, and unpredictable, because its variables are always changing.

Conversely, your general motivation to do things is remarkably simple and stable. While the momentary decision to eat a doughnut takes place *inside a particular context*, your general thoughts on consuming doughnuts are calculated *outside of context*. Your general motivation is your theoretical view. My general desire is to avoid eating doughnuts because they're unhealthy. That said, if you offered me $5,000 to eat a doughnut, I'd eat two.

When Your Perfect Ideals Fall off a Bridge
Isolated and without context, we would *always* make choices based on our general desires. But our strong, perfect ideals must first cross a rickety bridge known as Context to make it to the other side that we call Reality, and they don't always make it across.

When the doughnut is glazed so masterfully, you're hungry, and your friends are enjoying doughnuts of their own, suddenly your general desire to avoid eating doughnuts seems unimportant. It didn't make it across the bridge. Context can *easily* override our general desires, and this is the weakness of motivation-based strategies. They fail when "life happens."

Your general motivations in life are tied to your values and goals. These are your underlying *reasons* for your desired lifestyle, and they rarely change. Here's the problem: People tend to think, "My motivation (i.e., reason) not to eat cake will motivate me (i.e., give me the immediate desire) to not eat cake for dessert tonight." That would work, except that your general motivation is *not always strong enough* to defeat the other motivational influences you can't control. The first rule for living a good life is to focus on what you can control. As such, it's best to **separate** these two concepts into something we can control (general motivation) and something we can't fully control (momentary motivation).

When people talk about "getting and staying motivated," they're trying to control this wild mix of variables that are always changing. They think they can reliably cross the bridge of Context and bring their perfect ideals into real life. Depending on how you look at it, it's either hilarious or sad that so many people believe this. When your dog dies, when you are sick and exhausted, when you're tempted in just the right way, and when you're "just not feeling it," not only do you stand to lose the motivation battle, it might not even take place!

Isn't it interesting that the whole "get motivated" theory presupposes that we'll always *be motivated to get motivated*. What if we aren't? Do we then try to get motivated *to get motivated*? There is an easier way to go about this, but before we get to it, it's useful to know why we try to go through this process.

Why We Prefer Using Motivation to Willpower

This final point is important to understand: We like to use motivation to reach our goals, because being motivated to do something means you already want to do it. All things equal, doing what you want to do is preferable to forcing yourself to do things. When motivation is your guiding light, everything you do *feels right* (even when it isn't).

Nobody will *always* be motivated to do the right things, and that means trouble if you only act when motivated. What if an Olympic athlete only trained when (s)he felt like it? What if people only did their taxes when the IRS made them feel warm inside? What if people only showered when they were excited about it? The athlete would lose, the tax evaders would be punished, and the unmotivated showerers would smell terrible. They would all lose. Relying on motivation to take action is playing to lose, and that's why it's not a part of the *Mini Habits* strategy.

People will (correctly) say that motivation is necessary to do anything, even to lift your finger. This is why we separated the two types of motivation. You need to have a *reason* to act. No debate there. That's important. If you have no reason to do 17 jumping jacks right now, you won't do it. This, however, does NOT mean that your reason to do something must be stronger than all of your other contextual motivations. **If you have a good reason to do something but you don't want to do it, you can still do it.**

Momentary motivation is like turbo. It's fun when it's there, but don't use it as your primary fuel source. If not motivation, then what? Willpower.

Willpower

Let's try an exercise from *Mini Habits*. If I ask you to touch your nose right now, you will be able to do it. Your momentary motivation to do it is probably weak, because the only reason to do it is that I asked you to and you might want to experiment. You know that no tangible benefit will come from doing it. It's possibly annoying to consider doing something so trivial. And yet, if you decide to touch your nose, even if you are not motivated to do it, you still can.

You can act against your momentary motivation by using willpower. Willpower is a better starting point for action than motivation, because even if your Contextual bridge collapses and you're unmotivated, you still have the tools to cross that bridge. Using willpower means being prepared for the Contextual bridge to collapse. But could you force yourself to touch your nose 100 times in a row right now? Or 1,000 times? How about 30,000 times? Probably not, and that is the limit of willpower.

An effective strategy for all changes (especially one as challenging as weight loss) must enable you to succeed not only in ideal circumstances, but also in the *worst circumstances*. Willpower can work even when motivation is partially or completely lacking, but if it is to be our main strategy, we must explore its weaknesses.

Roy F. Baumeister of Florida State University could be called the father of willpower. Baumeister pioneered many of the dozens of experiments done to date that have shown that when we use willpower to do one thing, we lose some strength to use it for other things. Like a muscle, willpower has been shown to fatigue with use, and get stronger with training. This ego depletion model has been the predominant willpower theory in the last few decades. Over 200 studies have been performed to test and validate it.

A popular and oft-cited 2010 meta-analysis on ego depletion summarized the findings: "Significant effect sizes were found for ego depletion on effort, perceived difficulty, negative affect, subjective fatigue, and blood glucose levels."[25] These five areas were found to lower one's willpower strength in subsequent tasks, which makes them our biggest obstacles to consistent action with a willpower-first strategy. In *Mini Habits*, I discuss how each of these areas of weaknesses is mitigated or eliminated by the mini habits strategy.

Some researchers have questioned this ego depletion model, or the idea that willpower use is finite.[26] But the argument of whether or not our willpower will last forever or "deplete" is irrelevant. Since a good behavior change strategy must be able to succeed in the *worst* circumstances, it's best to design a strategy that works in low willpower situations.

Willpower Is Relative

Willpower is relative to actions. You can force yourself to touch your nose at any time, but how often can you force yourself to write a 450-page novel in one sitting? Against easy tasks, your willpower will seem sufficient if not strong. Against difficult tasks, your willpower will seem weak.

People tend to focus on the concept of "willpower reserves," as if the amount of "willpower in the tank" determines whether they succeed or fail. Do you see the folly in this mindset? Your baseline willpower at any given time is *much* less important than your goal. **While you may not be able to choose how much willpower you have, you can choose your goal, which determines your *relative willpower strength*.**

You don't need to worry about how willpower is depleted, if your willpower is depleted at any given time, or if it even can be. Instead, learn to succeed in all circumstances with mini habits. Mini habits work well in low motivation, low willpower, high motivation, and high willpower situations.

Mini Habits Maximize Success

The two most important scenarios for a human being are low willpower and high motivation situations. When your willpower is low, you want to avoid losing. When you're motivated, you want to maximize the opportunity to move forward. A mini habit thrives in both scenarios.

Mini habits are "forced actions" so small that even a willpower-depleted individual can still complete them. Unlike motivation-driven systems that require you to be "pumped up" in order to take "massive action," you can *crush* your mini habit goals on the worst day of your life (not just meet, *crush*). Think about how powerful that is. If you can still move forward on the worst day of your life, what can stop you? Even if an asteroid struck Earth, you'd continue to do your mini habits in the afterlife.

As for high motivation situations, a mini habit has no ceiling. You are encouraged to do more than your mini requirement (bonus reps). For example, if your mini habit is to meditate for one minute, you may continue to meditate for two hours if you wish.

Imagine being and feeling unstoppable when looking at a big change you want to make. It's different from what most people experience, because most advice is based on rising to the level of your intimidating goals. Most advice tells you that you have to become great just to be at eye level with your goals. On the day you're not feeling it, or on the day your pet parrot Picasso dies, your goals are going to tower over you in your down state, and you won't even attempt to look them in the eye. With a mini habit, it's different: you're always succeeding, always the stronger one, and always moving forward. In no area is frequent success and encouragement more important than weight loss!

Don't believe the books that tell you that you need to "want it more." Isn't it a bit insulting to tell a reader that they don't want something enough when they've bought your book in hopes to change that very thing? I think it is, which is why I don't doubt that you genuinely want to get healthier and look better. Many people *desperately* want to lose weight, and it's not their amount of desire that holds them back, it's their adoption of mainstream motivational strategies (and their prior experiences with them) that make them believe it can't actually be done. It can be done. Mini habits, smart strategies, and a small sliver of willpower are all you need.

3

Weight Loss Speed

Beware the Counterattack

"Be careful about reading health books. You may die of a misprint."
~ Mark Twain

Weight Gain Secrets

Since you're reading this book, I'm going to assume that you'd like to lose weight, but here's an interesting idea for you to think about. What if your goal was to *gain* fat? Bear with me here, because this is going to change the way you think about weight loss.

I'm getting at the fundamentals of change, because to gain fat is a body change just as much as losing fat is a body change. Thus, these two processes, while opposite in goal, share the fundamental component of changing from a previously established norm. How do people typically gain fat and become overweight?

Do they pump their fist at 12:01 AM on January 1st and say, "This is it. I'm really going to do it. I will gain 35 pounds this year!"?

Do they post to Facebook saying, "Hey everyone. I'm really serious about it this time. My goal is to gain 10 pounds this week on a milkshake cleanse."

Do they get inspired at 2 AM one night to consume more cheeseburgers, fries, and soda?

Do they swear to never leave the couch again?

All in all, do they stand on the proverbial mountain and declare the change that was about to happen?

Or does it just… happen? Gradually. Subtly. Sneakily. Pizza-ly.

People gain weight in the same way that people successfully lose weight: small and seemingly insignificant lifestyle choices accumulate over time into bigger changes. No matter what those "fast weight loss" books tell you, real change doesn't happen from a huge and sudden shift in behavior. The accumulation and progression of small changes is how we all change over time (without always intending to). It's how you've developed every bad habit you currently have, and though it's often a powerful force to our detriment, we can harness this same power for our benefit.

Your Body Does Not Want to Change

According to a 2006 Duke University Journal Study, the subconscious part of the brain dictates about 45% of our behavior in the form of habits.[27] As we covered, the subconscious mind is a routine-driven machine—it dislikes change and will resist it. This makes it the grim reaper of goal pursuits, because every goal pursuit is a change from your current position.

Beyond subconscious resistance, there is yet another layer to overcome— biological resistance. Weight loss experts refer to this as the body's "fat set point." The set point is the amount of fat the body currently holds and will try to maintain.

Mainstream weight loss strategies have us fight the fat set point, but not intelligently! The studies I mentioned earlier on calorie restriction and yo-yo dieting are a good example of *worsening* the fat set point by triggering the starvation response. The fat set point is so persistent that not even surgery can change it.

Surgical Fat Removal Doesn't Work

Liposuction is the surgical removal of fat from the body, and it doesn't work because of the fat set point. A study at the University of Colorado found that after one year, liposuction patients' body fat was no different from the control group.[28] Obesity researchers weren't surprised by this, as it's well known by now that our fat stores are controlled by the central nervous system.[29]

The most surprising thing is that liposuction remains popular. After breast augmentation and nose reshaping, liposuction was the third most popular cosmetic surgery procedure in the United States in 2014.[30] Not only that, but it was the only procedure in the top five to have registered an increase over the previous year.

As for how the body regains fat after surgical removal, it's likely as simple as increased food intake. A rat study (you want to hear more about rats? I knew it!) found that those that had fat tissue surgically removed ate more compared to the control group. "Over a wide range of body compositions, there was once again a clear inverse relationship between the induced change in adipose tissue mass and spontaneous chow intake."[31] Some may read this and think calorie counting could prevent the regain, but they'd be missing the point. This is yet another warning sign *against* aggressive plans like calorie restriction.

Dr. Salans, an obesity researcher at the Mount Sinai School of Medicine, says, "I suspect that the body's regulation of weight is so complex that if you intervene at this site, something else is going to happen to neutralize this intervention."[32]

The Human Body Demands Balance

Let's zoom out and take notice of a larger concept at work here. Balance. Here are just some of the ways the body fights for balance. Internalize the concept behind these facts and think about some of your previous extreme weight loss attempts in this context.

- When you consume insufficient sugar or carbohydrates, your body converts fat into glucose to maintain proper energy and bodily functioning. This is called ketosis.
- When you consume sugar or carbohydrates, your body produces an appropriate amount of insulin to uptake some of the glucose energy into cells and normalize your blood sugar levels.
- When you consume a lot of cholesterol, the liver makes less of it to compensate. When you consume less, the liver makes more. This is why high-cholesterol foods like eggs can still be very healthy (and not cause your cholesterol to rise).
- When blood is drawn, your body will produce a greater amount of red and white blood cells and platelets until levels are back to normal.
- When you exercise more (expend energy), you get hungrier (to intake energy).
- When you semi-starve yourself, your hormones will make you hungrier until you eat, and then you'll be more likely to overeat.
- When you semi-starve yourself and lose fat quickly, your body burns fewer calories at rest (food efficiency).
- When you process food and it's stored as fat, your fat cells will release the hormone leptin, which gives you the sensation of fullness. The amount of fat in your cells determines the amount of leptin released. Therefore, the more fat you have, the more leptin will be released, and the fuller you'll feel. This is a key way appetite is regulated (unless the person develops leptin resistance, which can block the "I have enough" signal).

Our bodies are machines of balance. Everything we know about the body shows a clear biological pattern of homeostasis, or the tendency to self-stabilize. This makes weight loss an interesting proposition, because the goal is to radically change something that doesn't want to change radically.

If you've gained fat, your body is fighting to keep it. Knowing this, is the smart approach to "shock" the body into a new way of living? Must we stop eating food completely for a while for the body to get the message? Of course not. This is like cornering a dangerous animal. If you do this to your body, you're going to provoke *its very best counterattack*. It's going to do whatever it can to get you back to your starting weight and may overcompensate to make you gain even more weight. It's like when the bank incorrectly shuts down your accounts "for your protection." It's frustrating, but the body is just doing its job.

Slow, Easy, Sneaky Changes

"Sure, I'll try a cigarette," said the chain smoker on the day that began a lifelong habit. "It's only 50 cents more to add chips and a drink?" said the man who didn't want to turn down a "good deal" and added 30 pounds of fat in the next two years as a result. If only we could use this technique to form good habits! We can.

Bad habits are easy to form because they are highly rewarding and easy to do. Good habits are difficult to form because the reward is delayed and *we make them hard to do*. The logical approach is to make bad habits harder to do and good habits easier to do.

Easy Does it

Have you ever gotten into a thermostat battle with someone? You're hot, so you move the temperature down three degrees. Someone else gets cold, and they move it back up three degrees and then a couple extra. Clever thermostat veterans win by changing it one degree at a time to avoid shocking cold-sensitive housemates into an overreaction.

Small changes don't trigger your body's "countermeasures." In *Mini Habits*, I discussed how small behavioral changes are subtle enough to avoid subconscious resistance (or at least lessen it considerably). Small dietary and fitness adjustments work the same way to avoid biological resistance. This is why mini habits—the kings of behavior change—are also the kings of weight loss.

Sneaky Does it

Fortunately or unfortunately, depending on your circumstances, your body is active tissue programmed to survive. After blatant calorie restriction, the body reacts as it should for survival—you more readily store fat from the food you eat.[33]

Losing weight is best approached as a covert operation. The change you want to reach is like a diamond in the center of a high security building. In this analogy, your body is the high security building, and fat is the diamond you wish to remove. Mainstream weight loss methods will tell you to run in the building with reckless abandon. And guess what? You'll get the diamond quickly! But what's this? You just set off 17 alarms, the building is in lockdown, the police have been notified, and a stressed-out security guard is pointing his gun at you. This is how your body responds to drastic weight loss measures.

You got the diamond (lost weight), but you'll have to put (gain) it back before you leave the building.

This analogy is not extreme; it is *exactly* what happens when people try to change rapidly. The body has built-in homeostasis "alarms" to prevent change. It goes by the motto of "If it ain't broke, don't (you dare try to) fix it." Your body says, "We've got a calorie deficit! Major calorie deficit! Send in the brownie lobbyists and set up a level four craving at noon!"

Your failure wasn't in obtaining the diamond (losing weight/fat); it was in having no exit strategy (lasting removal). Do you see how this also describes the dieting industry? They emphasize the fastest possible results, with little consideration given to what happens afterwards. Some people believe they can quickly lose weight and then go back to their former lifestyle without gaining it back. I wish it were true, but studies show that it's not. Others believe that a fast weight loss start will inspire them to do more, but, just like in long-distance races, extreme starts result in exhausted finishes.

Instead of running in recklessly to steal the diamond, a smarter thief would spend some time planning before entering the building. And what do you think the resulting strategy would be? The heist would be done at night. Slowly. Carefully. Surgically. Steadily. Sneakily. He'd move through the building while avoiding the sensors. Then, he'd claim the prize and escape. Nobody would know he was there.

If you can lose weight without triggering your body to overcorrect, the prize isn't just a lower number on the scale. The prize is changing your behavior permanently to support a new weight level and healthier body. That's worth more than any diamond.

When you use this approach, you also gain the benefits of compounding that we covered in the introduction. When you put it together, you have a reliable way to decrease your fat set point that can also compound into greater progress, more confidence, happiness, hope, and courage to continue forward. It's not just the best way, it is THE way to approach weight loss. Let's step out of theory now and get specific with the Mini Habits strategy.

The Mini Habits Strategy

Now that we've covered how the brain and body are best changed at their natural slow pace, I want to give you a condensed explanation of the mini habits strategy.

What *Exactly* Is a Mini Habit?
A mini habit is a "stupid small" behavior you do every day. I say "stupid small" because they sound absolutely ridiculous and generally take one minute or less to accomplish.

- One push-up a day
- Read two pages in a book per day
- Clean your home (or a specific area in it) for one minute per day
- Strike a key (on piano, guitar, etc.) or play one song per day
- Stretch one body part per day
- Eat one serving of fresh vegetables per day
- Floss one tooth per day

A mini habit doesn't look very useful on paper. Instinct is to say, "But I can do more than that!" And of course, we usually *can* do more than that. But the idea is to drop the requirement so low that "usually" becomes "always." When you can *always* do something, you're unstoppable. When you can *usually* do something, it means you're stoppable, and that isn't

43

good enough if you want lasting change. The best way to tell if your mini habit is too big is if you can't do it on your worst day. If you can succeed on the worst day(s) of your life, you won't fail.

In addition to doing this small behavior every day, you will also be encouraged to do what I call "bonus reps," which comes from the one push-up mini habit (the first one I had). A bonus rep is an additional repetition of your mini habit. So if your mini habit is to dance to one song every day, you might choose to dance to two or three songs on some days when you feel especially groovy, or perhaps dance for a few more seconds after the song is over. If your mini habit is to eat a serving of fresh vegetables at lunch, maybe one day you'll have two servings at lunch, or an additional serving at dinner. Bonus reps are anything extra, and there's no amount too small or too large. My 50 words of writing per day mini habit has sometimes expanded to 100 words or exploded into 5,000 words. Both are bonuses. Both are great!

Bonus reps are always optional, never required. You are always permitted to do your mini habit and stop there because a mini habit *must* stay small. Even if you've done bonus reps for 57 days in a row, you can always stop at the mini habit. A low requirement and high ceiling is perfect for consistency plus unlimited upward potential.

The mini habit is the base of our strategy. It ensures that you'll develop a new habit (that will benefit you for a lifetime). The bonus reps are an outlet for any excess motivation or grit that you may have on a given day. This system *adapts to you* on a daily basis.

Every other plan you'll come across presents you with a flat, high target. For example, a traditional nutrition-based diet includes a list of foods you are allowed to eat and some that you aren't. If you're lucky, you will get a single cheat day per week. But what if you don't need a cheat day? What if you need two? You have to adapt to it, rather than it to you.

The traditional structure of weight loss programs pressures you to rise to the challenge every day, and on the days you're not able to do it, you will feel defeated and like a failure. Dieting probably has the highest quitting rate of any pursuit, which says a lot about it and little about the people who try it.

In traditional goal pursuit, the beginning marks the highest point of motivation. It is slowly drained as time goes on, and practically destroyed once the first failure occurs. The mini habits strategy is the opposite. It's rooted in positivity and designed for almost certain success every day. When you succeed every day, your confidence, self-efficacy, and motivation won't shrink over time; they will grow.

4

Everyone's Wrong

Weight Loss Is Not about Carbs, Fat, or Calories

*"What you eat actually changes how you expend energy.
Similarly, how you expend energy changes what (and how) you
eat. To be even more nuanced, what you eat further impacts
what you subsequently eat. As you increase (or decrease) in
size, this impacts how you expend energy."*[34]
~ Peter Attia, MD

Setting the Terms

Now that we've talked about brain change and body change, it's time to discuss nutrition. This is the science-y discussion about how weight loss works. In this chapter, we'll be seeking to answer the question of "What's the best way to lose weight?" Before we get into that, I must clarify something.

Observations Are Not Recommendations
I'm going to be talking about how weight loss works, and that means I'll say or imply things such as "processed food causes weight gain." Most people (and authors) will immediately assume that the statement "processed food causes weight gain" means the answer is to "forbid processed food." This is not smart.

Strategy is our best weapon, and forbidding something is only one possible strategy of *many* to reach the goal of losing weight. Forbidding food is the dumbest strategy you can employ because it plays to our weakness (we'll discuss why in depth later).

"Ultra-Processed" Foods
I'm going to refer to processed foods often in this chapter. Technically, all foods are processed on some level. Fruits and vegetables are often rinsed before sold, and even that is considered a form of processing. Animal meat is processed on wildly varying levels (a rotisserie chicken is far less processed than a hot dog). In this book, when I say "processed foods," I'm really referring to ultra-processed foods, which are defined below by Carlos Monteiro, PhD, MD.

"Ultra-processing is used to make products from combinations of ingredients extracted from whole foods, usually with little or even no whole foods. Typically, series of processes are used, in the creation of the ingredients and also in the creation of the products, which also usually contain some or many preservatives and cosmetic additives. They are formulated to be hyper-palatable, of long duration, and are usually packaged ready to consume. They are very profitable, and aggressively marketed. They are the end product of a chain of processes."

Food Comparisons
To make all of the upcoming comparisons and examples simple, I'm going to use 100 grams as the base amount of food.[35] The weight of food

is fascinating in how it relates to its calorie content. You'll see why eating fruits and vegetables lead you to eating significantly fewer calories. The numbers are shocking.

Simple as Possible, Not Simpler

"Everything should be made as simple as possible, but not simpler."
~ Albert Einstein

One of the greatest problems in the weight loss industry is oversimplified claims. The following claims may be true in certain circumstances, but not as blanket statements:

- "Carbs make us fat."
- "Calories in, calories out."
- "Fat makes us fat."

These popular explanations for human weight gain and loss are simple. Unfortunately, they violate Einstein's rule above because they are *simpler* explanations than necessary. The biological mechanisms of weight are extraordinarily complex, and while they can be simplified to an applicable degree, these are (way) too simple to be accurate.

You can only come up with simple, true, and effective solutions if you thoroughly understand the problem, which is why this is a book and not a one liner—"Hey, just take small steps to weight loss!" Great depth of research and analysis went into the *Mini Habits for Weight Loss* strategy.

The Process of Getting to Effective and Simple Solutions
When we have a basic, but not masterful, understanding of a challenge, we come up with complicated solutions, as beautifully captured in this quote:

"I would have written a shorter letter, but I did not have the time."
~ Blaise Pascal

Simple, concise, and effective solutions take the most time and effort to create. Computers are a great example—one computer used to take up an entire room! Computer programming started on physical "punch cards." In order to tell the room-sized computer what to do, you'd mark the cards in particular spots and make a deck to feed into the computer. Our computing solution was cumbersome and complicated because we hadn't yet mastered the technology.

As our understanding of technology has improved, so have computers. They are many multitudes smaller, more powerful, more intuitive, and easier to use and understand. The masterful depth of understanding we've gained for this technology has made computers easier to use.

As understanding improves, solutions get closer to Einstein's "simple as possible" ideal. But if understanding is wrong altogether, people will create solutions that seem to be simple and correct, but they're often *simpler than necessary and therefore incorrect*, and that's what we have in the weight loss industry. Obesity rates have gotten worse despite the research and money we've thrown at it, which suggests that we haven't improved our understanding of the problem.

"Carbs make us fat"

If carbs make us fat, then why was a Harvard professor able to lose 27 pounds on a diet of carb-heavy processed food for two months (famously called "The Twinkie Diet")? Why do so many cultures remain lean with high-carb diets? It doesn't take much to discredit this idea, because carbohydrates have been eaten for thousands of years without associated weight issues.

And yet, low-carb diets appear to be fairly successful for weight loss in the short term (when adhered to). Do carbs make us fat or not? That's the wrong question, because the concept of "carbs make us fat" is simpler than necessary.

"Calories in, Calories out"

If counting calories is the answer, why does traditional calorie counting math suggest we should all weigh over 900 pounds by now?[36] What about the proven role of hormones to moderate food intake over the long term? What about the "fat set point," which is governed by the central nervous system, not by how many 100-calorie snack packs you eat?

And of course, if only calories matter, why do many studies (that we discussed in the introduction) provide compelling evidence that restricting calories now makes us gain even more weight later? Calorie restriction has been shown to drop your metabolism and make your body prone to store fat.

The amount of calories we consume obviously matters some and plays a role in weight management. But do calorie surpluses make us fat and calorie deficits make us thin? That's the wrong question, because the concept of "calories in, calories out" is simpler than necessary.

"Fat Makes Us Fat"

If fat makes us fat, then why does coconut oil (as fatty as a fat can be, and mostly saturated!) appear to reduce abdominal fat and aid weight loss efforts?[37] Why do many high-fat diets lead to weight loss? If fat is *the* reason behind weight loss, then high-fat diets should make weight loss impossible, but they seem to do the opposite in many cases.

And yet, fat is generally less satiating, contains more calories per gram, and can be eaten in higher quantities than carbs or protein. Does fat make us fat or not? That's the wrong question, because the concept of "fat makes us fat" is simpler than necessary.

These explanations don't account for the big picture. There are many ways to lose weight in the short term, meaning even the worst ideas (see Twinkie diet) can be "validated." The Twinkie diet didn't prove that only calories matter: it showed that you can probably lose weight in two months if you don't eat enough food. We already knew that. Sustainability matters unless you only care about weight loss in the summer.

Non-Calorie Weight Loss Factors

The dietary factors that regulate weight include: food nutrition, calorie density, insulin resistance, leptin resistance, inflammation, genetic disposition to weight gain, food satiety, and food satisfaction (i.e., the hedonic reward system). This doesn't mean the solutions are complex—don't forget this is a book about doing easy mini habits—it only means that calorie counting is wrong because it says that *only* calories matter. The amount of calories we eat does matter, but it's not all that matters and it does not matter most.

The first law of thermodynamics states that energy can transfer to a different form, but it cannot be created or destroyed. Applied to our bodies, if you take in more energy than you expel, then you will weigh more. This is obvious, like saying that a room full of puppies has fewer puppies in it if some puppies leave the room. When it comes to the weight battle, the key question is what strategy makes your fat "leave the room" for good.

The obvious solution so many people try is to eat fewer calories and burn more to create a deficit. This works in the short term, but feeling hungry all the time and wrecking your metabolism isn't a permanent solution, is it? Even if you were willing to remain hungry all of the time to be thinner, it would be a constant temptation and frustration; only willpower superheroes win that war.

Besides, calorie restriction has far worse consequences than mere hunger. In the introduction, we covered studies showing that extended calorie restriction caused an alarming propensity for *weight gain* in rats and humans. (If you know any rats, please let them know about these studies.) In the Minnesota Starvation Experiment, one of the primary observations was that most of the men became depressed and emotionally distressed from eating too few calories.[38] The body isn't meant to change this way, and it reacts accordingly. Our goal isn't to stop eating so much food (calorie counting); it's to figure out *why* we eat too much food—on a biological and emotional level—and how to reverse that.

The Truth about Weight Loss

Food can be separated into three groups: whole foods, ultra-processed foods, and everything in-between. The simple as possible (but not simpler than necessary) truth about weight loss is that ultra-processed foods are the primary reason why we gain weight and fail to lose it.

Ultra-processed foods can be further broken down into carbs, fats, or calories, but at that point, we run into problems. It's not any one of those factors that make processed foods weight-gaining—it's all of them, plus a lack of nutrition, inflammatory ingredients, and poor satiety. Thus, we can't go any simpler than "ultra-processed foods cause weight gain" and "unprocessed whole foods aid weight loss." When you look at the calories or macronutrients of processed food and draw overarching conclusions (as many have done), you incorrectly include many healthy, weight-friendly foods that happen to be high in fat, calories, or carbs.

Let's talk about macronutrients, and then calories.

Macronutrient Wars

Many weight loss discussions today revolve around macronutrients (carbs, fat, and protein). For example, The American Heart Association has been recommending a low-fat diet for many years. This is terrible. Here's how it started.

In the middle of the 20th century, scientists were in a frenzy to find the reason for the rapid increase of obesity and heart disease rates in the USA. Then, in 1955, United States President Dwight Eisenhower suffered a left anterior myocardial infarction (i.e., a heart attack). This amplified that frenzy.

Nutritionist Ancel Keys led us to the door of dietary fat as the culprit of the problem, because he studied seven countries' dietary habits and heart disease statistics. His data showed a trend of fat consumption correlating with heart disease. Some say that he only picked the countries which supported his hypothesis, and left out countries like Norway, where the diet is high in fat but heart disease is low, or Chile, where the diet is low in fat but heart disease is high.

Nevertheless, the low-fat revolution was born. The food industry loved it because they had a brilliant new marketing angle: low-fat foods. They had just one problem: fat makes food taste better. In order to offset the poorer taste of low-fat foods, they added more sugar. They solved the taste problem, and made everyone fatter in the process. In recent years, people have warmed up to the idea that fat isn't all bad, and sugar (and carbohydrates in general) have been under intense scrutiny from various experts and new diets.

Too few recognize the broader issue of focusing on macronutrients. Many have gone from demonizing fats to demonizing carbohydrates. We now have one battle of fats vs. carbs and a separate battle of macronutrients vs. calories. These are both the wrong battles!

Between fats and carbs, which one is the cause of weight gain and the preventer of weight loss? Neither. There are good and bad fats for weight loss, and there are good and bad carbs for weight loss.

Macronutrients are not the problem or the solution. That philosophy equates a boiled potato to a French fry to a pile of sugar to brown rice because "they're carbs." It equates coconut oil to lard to trans fat to saturated fat to unsaturated fat to soybean oil to fish oil because "they're fats." It's nonsense.

I'm Not a Conspiracy Theorist, but...

What would be the result be—and for the record, I say this semi-jokingly and to provoke some thoughts—if the processed food industry could manipulate the obesity argument to change from healthy vs. unhealthy food to a macronutrient or calorie debate?

The processed food industry is cunning. If they are somehow behind this macronutrient focus, they are not just cunning, they're (evil) geniuses. The way they design and meticulously test food to be addictive in texture, flavor, and taste is impressive, but to manipulate how we see weight loss to sustain robust sales would be a they-should-make-a-movie-out-of-this level of corrupt brilliance.

As with calorie counting, a focus on macronutrients changes "processed food" to just food. It simplifies food into carbs, fat, and protein, and all foods, processed and unprocessed, contain those. Basically, when macronutrients are the focus, there's no distinction between processed and unprocessed foods.

If the only difference between an avocado and a fat-free cupcake is that they have different macronutrient profiles, we can eat whichever one fits our diet better. Or better yet, since cupcakes are so delightful, we could choose *what specialized type of cupcake* we want without the consequences of whatever macronutrient we believe is evil at the time. Food scientists could create low-fat cupcakes, sugar-free cupcakes, low-sodium cupcakes, and gluten-free cupcakes, and, by appealing to so many different macronutrient-based diets, it would translate into more products, more sales, and more revenue. (And yes, all of those cupcake varieties actually exist.)

What's the only motivator more powerful than desire? Fear. People's fear of fat would lead them to select fat-free yogurt (that's loaded with sugar). If it's carbs they fear, they'd buy artificially sweetened desserts instead of "scary" whole fruit with natural fructose. The only thing more lucrative than a person eating a regular cupcake for pleasure is a person eating a specialized type of cupcake out of fear.

A widespread focus on macronutrients combined with modified foods is the ultimate fear weapon to provoke sales in more food niches. Since processed food is created in labs and produced in factories, it can be manipulated to have any macronutrient profile the scientists desire. Take out the fat? No problem. Take out the sugar? Easy. Take out the sodium? Done. Natural food, on the other hand, can't morph like that. A blueberry, one of the most effective weight loss foods in the world, will always contain some sugar (fructose).

Is it just a coincidence that the prevailing theories give processed food such a significant advantage over natural foods? It's possibly coincidence, but look at the data on obesity. You will see in numerous studies that processed food's fingerprints are all over the obesity crime scene, with millions dead and billions currently overweight with associated health problems. It makes you wonder *why else* we'd still be looking at macronutrients. Even though the meteoric rise of processed food has coincided with the meteoric rise in obesity worldwide (like a pair of synchronized swimmers), too many people are *still* focused on "fats and carbs."

Consider this: fats and carbs have both been eaten as long as food has existed. (That's a long time.) Common sense has to play a role in the debate about what's really causing obesity. Obesity didn't skyrocket when carbs and fat were introduced; it skyrocketed when these *new kinds* of ultra-processed carbs and fat were introduced.

Asian cultures have traditionally eaten a very high carbohydrate diet (with lots of white, carbtastic rice), and they've remained fit and healthy overall. White rice is nutritionally inferior to brown rice, but it is still a one-ingredient food. Scandinavian countries have low death rates and relatively low obesity rates, and eat a high fat diet. It's not because they eat fat or carbs; it's because the fat and carbs they eat most often are better quality than countries with widespread obesity.

Speaking of quality, let's talk about calories, where quantity is a common, but incorrect focal point.

The Inequality of Calories

Every calorie you consume has a unique hormonal and metabolic impact in your body. Two foods of the same caloric value are different in biological satisfaction, perceived satisfaction, satiety, insulin response, nutrient content (which affects the health and function of our organs), and energy distribution, all of which can impact your behavior and weight in the short and long term. With the "calories in, calories out" (CICO) way of thinking, these factors are considered irrelevant, even though they *will* affect your food decisions, including how many calories you feel compelled to eat.

To be clear, overeating the right foods could potentially cause weight gain —it's possible—but it's challenging to do because of their typically high satiety-to-calorie ratio, nutritional value, and body-healing compounds. Also, let's not only deal in extremes. The goal isn't to *overstuff* ourselves while eating the right foods. Hunger levels span from hungry to satiated to full to "belt-snapping." The goal is smooth and consistent satiety, not bouncing from extreme calorie restriction to bingeing (yo-yo dieting). If we eat good food to satiety, we can lose weight, feel satisfied, and not have to deal with the issues that arise from undereating.

The Mango Binge

One night, I ate an entire 10 ounce (284g) bag of sliced frozen mangoes. It was a lot of fruit, and it was delicious. I thought, "I really overdid it," until I looked at the bag and saw I had eaten only 200 calories! A single 52.7g Snickers bar contains 250 calories. The bag of mangoes is more than five times heavier than the Snicker's bar, and yet the bar still has 25% more calories!

You can't just blame the calorie difference on the higher fat content in the Snicker's bar, either. Avocados get 82% of their calories from fat, and yet a 150g serving of avocado only amounts to 240 calories, which makes it three times heavier, almost all fat, and *still* fewer calories than a Snicker's bar. The difference is due to calorie density and water content. Psychologically, it might feel more indulgent to eat an entire 10 ounce bag of mangoes than a single candy bar, but it's fewer calories and more nutrients.

Aside from the hassle of counting calories to make sure you starve yourself precisely, it's unnecessary. Whole foods will always possess the greatest satiety-to-calorie ratio, meaning there's no need to count calories if you eat the right foods. (If you think zero-calorie "diet foods" possess the greatest satiety-to-calorie ratio, you aren't considering their medium- and long-term effects on appetite.)

Calorie counting has become the most popular way to pretend unhealthy eating is a viable path to weight loss. They say you can eat junk food as long as it's below your calorie requirement. Since processed food is typically high calorie and not satiating, people who count calories as a means to justify a poor diet may end up semi-starved at the end of the day, and semi-starvation diets end in weight gain.

Calorie counting is like landing a cheap shot on a bigger and stronger fighter. You may catch him off guard and stun him for a moment, but once he regains his composure and figures out what's going on, you're toast.

Tracking how much food you eat, mindfulness, and eating in moderation are redeeming aspects of calorie counting, but the associated notion of all calories being equal is so inaccurate and devastating to progress that we need to throw the whole concept away. You can practice eating in moderation without counting calories. Satiety is nature's way of counting calories for you.

Satiety

Satiety is the feeling of being satisfied; in laymen's terms, it's not being hungry and having little to no desire to eat food.

Satiety collapses the calorie-counting argument by itself, because if calorie counting were the answer, the number of calories we ate would directly correlate to how full and satiated we felt. But that's not the case. Some foods actually *stoke* our hunger while others satiate us. Calorie counting fails because it doesn't consider satiety, and if you're chronically not satiated and have access to food, you'll make up the calorie deficit eventually (I'd put money on it)!

One could argue that satiety is most important in weight loss, because if you eat food that leads to weight loss and you're completely satisfied on a biological level, you have a good chance to win the fight in the long term. There are other factors that affect our food consumption, but the first, most basic goal to get right is satiety. How can we feel full and satisfied with what we eat AND lose weight? Is that even possible? Yes, and you'll see why with a few examples.

Since it's difficult to measure satiety directly and technically, we can use the mass of food as a starting point, since part of satiety is dictated by how much space food takes up in your stomach. This is the concept behind bariatric surgery, which makes your stomach much smaller so that you feel full faster and don't eat as much food. A safer alternative to surgically making your stomach smaller is to eat food that fills you up on fewer calories. Just for fun, let's compare some foods' calorie content to their mass. This will give you an idea of how much more satiating natural foods are.

Count *These* Calories

Half of a standard 8 oz bag of chips weighs about 100g and contains 536 calories. While that's a lot of chips, it's not difficult to eat that many in one sitting. Despite their high calorie content, chips do a poor job of making you feel full, and studies suggest that such high-fat, high-carb, high-energy processed foods may even trigger us to eat more food.[39]

Instead of that 100g half-bag of chips, you could eat 224g of chicken, which is highly satiating and more than twice as much food as the chips. You could *try* to eat 483g of brown rice (more than one pound). Or how about broccoli? Oh, I don't think you're ready for broccoli. If you thought chicken and rice were extreme compared to chips, this is going to stun you.

Instead of half a bag of chips, you could eat 1,000g (2.2 pounds) of broccoli for the same number of calories. I'm kidding. It's not 1,000g of broccoli, but not because it's too high. It's too low! That massive amount of broccoli—more than ten times the weight of the chips—is still not even close to the calorie content in half a bag of chips; 1,000g of broccoli would only set you back 340 calories! To eat enough broccoli to equal the number of calories in half a bag of chips, you'd have to eat 1,576g of it. That's right, *3.5 pounds* of broccoli is equivalent in calories to half a bag of chips. Good luck trying to eat that much broccoli in five days, let alone one session.

What about strawberries? To equal the amount of calories in half a bag of chips, you'd have to eat *3.6 pounds* of strawberries (1,624 grams). That means for a full bag of chips or a typical fast food meal,[40] the equivalent calorie value would be 7.2 pounds of strawberries. I'm not making this up. This information is available on the USDA website for anyone to see.

But it's the sugar in strawberries that's problematic, right? Eh, not really, as 3.6 pounds of strawberries only contains 79.6 grams of sugar. That's much less than one 32 oz soda, and you'd have to eat 3.6 pounds of them to consume that much sugar.

CICO teaches you to think, "Oh, this small bag of chips is only 160 calories." It's a flawed perspective, because it throws processed food into the discussion as a viable option for weight loss, when it is the primary cause of the global obesity epidemic. When it comes to bang for your calorie buck, you won't beat natural foods (and we'll talk about low-calorie processed foods soon).

Many would agree that the single worst part of dieting and calorie counting is hunger. But if you eat the right foods, you can *easily* eat fewer calories without feeling hungry. A 2016 study found "the more food is processed, the higher the glycemic response and the lower its satiety potential."[41]

For breakfast, I'll sometimes eat three hard-boiled eggs (150g) and drink water. It's quite filling for a small breakfast eater like me. At 78 calories per egg, I don't exceed 250 calories at breakfast. A 2008 study found that an egg breakfast enhanced weight loss, with a 61% greater reduction in BMI (Body Mass Index) than a group that ate bagels for breakfast.[42]

We don't need studies to tell us that eggs are satiating per calorie; we can also deduce that from the fact that they are a single ingredient, minimally processed food.

The Satiety Deception
We deceive ourselves when we compare the size of processed food and whole foods and conclude that "whole foods aren't as filling." This is exactly the opposite of the truth. *Whole foods are many times more filling than processed foods per calorie.*

"I'd eat salads, but I'm still hungry afterwards." I'm sure you've heard or said this statement before. Here's the problem: that salad you just ate is probably about 20% of the calories of your typical meal. That's like saying, "I'd eat one taco instead of three tacos, but it's not as filling." If you're hungry, you didn't eat enough. Eat more salad or other food if you're still hungry.

"Stuffing yourself" on healthy food still results in a low-calorie meal. A study found the average restaurant meal contained 1,327 calories.[43] Let's see what kind of healthy meal we could create with that many calories.

Half a pound of chicken (227g): 542 calories
One pound of boiled potatoes (454g): 395 calories
Two pounds of spinach (907g): 209 calories
Three pounds of green leaf lettuce (1,360g): 204 calories
Total from 6.5 pounds of food (2,948g): 1,350 calories

Okay, so we went slightly over the average calorie content of a restaurant meal. Oh, but this is 6.5 pounds of food. You don't need to fear overeating or being hungry if you're eating truly healthy foods. I even included some (relatively) high-calorie foods like chicken and potatoes, but these foods make up for it in satiety. Potatoes ranked as the most satiating food in the satiety index.[44]

Don't misinterpret this data. Almost all natural foods have a significantly higher satiety-per-calorie ratio over processed foods, which naturally leads to fewer calories eaten, but that's not the full story. We're not trading "only calories matter" for "only satiety-per-calorie matters." Satiety-per-calorie matters *more* than just calories, but high-fat, high-calorie natural foods can still be fantastic for weight loss for other reasons.

Only two tablespoons of olive oil (27g) is a whopping 238 calories (a calorie counter's nightmare). In a study of 28 women, 80% lost more than five pounds on an olive-oil enriched diet, compared to only 31% on a low-fat diet.[45] How could that be? Let's discuss the *other* factors that make unprocessed food great for weight loss.

The Supreme Importance of Unprocessed Food for Weight Loss

Unprocessed, natural, real food is essential for weight loss, and I know you've heard that before, but I'm going to explain some of the biological reasons why that is. These factors affect weight regulation, and they have nothing to do with calorie content.

Inflammation
Inflammation is not a bad thing that happens to us. It's our body's response to something bad that has *already* happened, such as infection or

injury. It's the body's way of fighting invaders or healing damaged tissue. When you sprain your ankle (and I've sprained each of mine several times playing basketball), blood flow to the ankle increases as white blood cells and other immune cells rush in to repair the damage, causing it to swell. Auto-immune problems (such as allergies) cause inflammation because the body thinks it needs to attack something that need not be attacked. It's like punching yourself in the face, but inside your body.

Obesity is an inflammatory disease.[46] This is basic scientific observation: Overweight people consistently show higher levels of systemic inflammation.[47] "This may explain the increased risk of diabetes, heart disease, and many other chronic diseases in the obese."[48]

Does inflammation cause obesity or the other way around? Inflammation and obesity fuel each other, so it's not a question of which comes first; it's a question of how to break the cycle.

Inflammation sustains the cycle. It interferes with leptin signals (the hormone secreted by fat cells to signal fullness to the brain), which lessens the satiety response from eating. In most overweight and obese people, leptin levels in the blood remain high, and yet the "I'm full" message doesn't get through. This is called leptin resistance, and it has been a key focal point for obesity researchers in the last 10-20 years. Scientists have found that "plasma levels of leptin and inflammatory markers are correlated,"[49] and "leptin production is acutely increased during infection and inflammation."[50]

If inflammation directly and/or indirectly impairs leptin sensitivity (which appears to be the case), it may be a major cause of obesity. If an individual doesn't know when to stop eating, that's a problem.

This is a big strike against processed foods, which contain inflammatory ingredients in the form of added flavors, colors, fats, emulsifiers, sweeteners, and preservatives.

A 2015 study found that emulsifiers are linked to obesity and gut disease by altering gut bacteria and causing inflammation in mice.[51] Trans fats have been linked to systemic inflammation in women.[52] Food coloring studies have shown that they're toxic to animals.[53] About a dozen food coloring chemical concoctions have already been banned by the FDA because of their toxicity (it makes you wonder if the current ones are really okay). Omega 6 fatty acids most commonly exist as various vegetable oils (such as soybean oil) in processed foods, and too many omega 6 fatty acids in relation to omega 3 fatty acids is linked to inflammation (and a host of diseases).[54]

Monosodium glutamate (MSG), a flavor enhancer commonly found in chips, crackers, and restaurant food, causes significant inflammation in rats.[55]

The excessive amount of sugar in processed foods causes inflammation, too. Nutritionist Julie Daniluk explained to CNN, "High amounts of sugar in the diet increase advanced glycation end-products, or AGEs, a protein bound to a glucose molecule, resulting in damaged, cross-linked proteins. As the body tries to break these AGEs apart, immune cells secrete inflammatory messengers called cytokines."[56]

The same goes for refined carbohydrates like white bread, pizza, burger buns, and most cereals, which are rapidly turned to glucose and sent into the bloodstream. The problem with refined grains is once again the processing, which basically "takes the life out" of the food. It strips out the nutrients and breaks down the food, making it more like an injection of glucose than something you need to digest.

In a single processed food, there are likely to be multiple inflammation-causing ingredients. Don't become numb to buzzwords such as MSG or trans fats just because "health nuts" talk about them. There is a lot of evidence that these substances are actually toxic to us. The chronic inflammation processed foods cause might not knock us on our backs instantly, but it will covertly make us fat, sick, and unhealthy. It's a double whammy, too, because the unprocessed fruits and vegetables we could be eating instead are full of anti-inflammatory compounds.

When you choose to eat that candy bar with artificial flavors, colors, and emulsifiers instead of a delicious mango, not only have you consumed several inflammatory ingredients, you missed out on powerful anti-inflammatory compounds.

Vitamins, Minerals, and Flavonoids

Natural, whole foods are full of bioavailable micronutrients that enable the entire body to work better. The more food is processed, the more such micronutrients are destroyed.

Can't you just take a multivitamin? That could help replace some of the nutrients missing from a diet rich in fruits and vegetables, but the nutrients in a multivitamin have varying levels of bioavailability (how well your body is able to absorb and use a substance).

Many vitamins you buy at the store are synthetically made, rather than derived from food. That's not automatically bad, but it does raise additional questions about their quality and suitability. Compare an artificial "orange drink" fortified with vitamin C to a vitamin C tablet to eating an orange. Even if, for argument's sake, you manage to absorb the vitamin C from the drink or tablet, you're still missing out on the flavonoids, enzymes, and minerals you'd get from a real orange. You're also missing the synergy!

Registered dietician Jackie Elnahar says, "When you remove a vitamin part from the whole food form, you get fractionated pieces of the whole, but that has consequences. Nature intended for you to consume food in WHOLE form, because all the vitamins, minerals, antioxidants, and enzymes together work synergistically to give your body the nutrition it requires for optimal health. Your body only absorbs a small percentage of an isolated form of a vitamin and/or mineral, and it utilizes even less, so the bioavailability is greatly affected. You get the best bioavailability in whole food form."[57]

Water Content

Most fruits and vegetables consist of over 80% water, and many of them are more than 90% water (cucumbers, tomatoes, watermelon, strawberries, broccoli, lettuce, etc.)! Because of their water content, fruits and vegetables are voluminous, filling, and low calorie.

In contrast, many processed foods have the opposite profile of a fruit or vegetable, some being less than 10% water. Less water content in food means it is less filling and less hydrating. If your goal is to consume more calories and gain weight, then processed food is the answer. Otherwise, whole foods are the way to lose weight.

What Happened When Sweden Ate More Processed Food

In a nationwide analysis of Sweden that covered 50 years (1960-2010), their consumption of unprocessed foods (fruits, vegetables, etc.) decreased 2%, and their consumption of "ultra-processed" food increased by 142%. *One hundred and forty-two percent.* In particular, soda (315% increase) and crisps/candies (367% increase) became much more popular. Sweden's obesity rate from 1980 to 2010 more than doubled, from 5% to 11%.[58] Are you surprised? I didn't mention fats, carbs, or calories. I just told you they ate a higher percentage of processed foods.

I know that "correlation is not causation," because two completely unrelated variables can correlate. The birth rate of turkeys may coincide perfectly with the number of milkshakes consumed in Arizona, but that doesn't mean one is causing the other. When a particular diet correlates with a change in weight, however, that's a different story, because we know diet affects weight. Sweden's increased consumption of processed food *is indeed* a major cause of rising obesity rates in their country. You could say it's the calories from these foods, because processed food is very calorie-dense. You could say it's the high-carb and/or high-fat profile of these foods, which have each been linked to overeating. But why overcomplicate such a clear and simple truth? It's processed foods.

When you say it's calories, it allows crafty corporations to create low-calorie ultra-processed foods that disrupt our hormones and trigger cravings. When you say it's fat, well, we've already tried that one, and the low-fat, processed-food revolution made everyone even fatter. When you say it's carbs, this eliminates most of the problematic processed foods, but it also eliminates a lot of great whole foods, and puts some awful, weight-gaining foods with artificial sweeteners on the highest pedestal. But when you say it's ultra-processed foods, you target *all* of the stuff that's made us fat over the last century, while sparing healthy food that we ate before obesity rates became extreme.

Not only is our macronutrient obsession too broad to be useful, but it's highly restrictive of the wrong foods and it's difficult to maintain. I have no "healthy granola bar" to sell you, so I have no reason to sugar-coat the truth, which is that there are almost no healthy granola bars.

The Role of Genetics

The reason some people have a diet high in processed foods and remain thin is genetics, just like those who eat a healthy diet and remain overweight. These people are a small portion of the population.

Seventy percent of Americans are overweight, but the American diet suggests that genetics play a small role. A nationally-representative cross-sectional study in the United States published in March 2016 found that "ultra-processed foods comprised 57.9% of the USA's total energy intake."[59] According to this data, I'd guess that 20% of Americans are actually *genetically predisposed to staying thin*, and the rest of us who are eating weight-gaining foods are gaining weight *as one would expect*.

Data like the Swedish analysis, the fact that obesity follows the Western diet around like a puppy, and the constant correlation between processed food consumption and obesity make it hard not to believe that processed food *isn't* behind it all. Saying anything other than "it's processed food" gives food corporations enough wiggle room to design their food to be part of a "healthy diet." It's time to stop the madness.

The determining factor of food quality is the degree to which it is processed. Avocados are 82% fat and don't make you fat. Fruit has sugar and doesn't make you fat. You can make an avocado more fattening by making it into guacamole with additives like salt and sugar, but don't blame the avocado. You can order a berry smoothie from a chain restaurant with added sugar or syrup, but don't blame the berries. You can drench a healthy salad in sugary soybean oil dressing, but don't blame the lettuce.

The reason we've targeted fats and carbs is because there *are* some terrible ones out there that do make us fat. The ones to be avoided exist exclusively in processed foods.

Follow the Money

Obesity rates are still climbing—[60]and we have more "healthy options" in processed food. Just look at the shelves. We have *organic* processed food in rustic, earth-toned packaging. We have naturally sweetened soda. In other words, we can choose "healthier" ways to gain weight. Hooray?

If it's so obvious that processed foods are hurting so many people, why won't companies just shift to marketing and selling whole foods? Money. Corporations exist to make a profit, and if they can make food that is attractive, delicious, addictive, cheap to manufacture, and in high demand, why wouldn't they? The United States is the worldwide capital of processed food *because we're so commerce-driven*. As a general rule, the more processed a food is, the more profitable it is.

Subsidized Crops Increase Profitability

The government supplements the income of farmers who grow certain crops. This ramps up the supply of these crops and drives down the price. Farmers have a greater financial incentive to produce a subsidized crop than a non-subsidized one.

In the United States, three of the main subsidized crops are corn, soybeans, and wheat. Not coincidentally, it's nearly impossible to find processed food that doesn't contain one of these ingredients. Almost every ultra-processed food contains soy, corn, and/or wheat ingredients. Did you know that *hundreds* of common ingredients are derived from corn, soy, and wheat? The documentary *King Corn* explores the role of corn in the United States, and how it is in almost everything we eat. If we just ate corn on the cob, maybe we'd be fine, but corn-derived ingredients affect your body differently than real corn.

Did You Know That Soybean Oil Has Taken Over?

In the 1940s, soybean oil was "considered neither a good industrial paint oil nor a good edible oil,"[61] and now it's everywhere. Of all oils consumed by Americans, 80% is soybean oil—80% of all oil consumed in the United States!

Do you know anyone who cooks at home with soybean oil? Me neither. But if you look at the ingredients of any processed food, you're sure to find soybean oil. At an organic grocery store, I could not find salad dressing made without soybean oil, so I had to buy olive oil and vinegar separately to use as dressing.

Many other vegetables oils were introduced in the 1900s, but since soybeans are a subsidized crop, soybean oil has become the go-to oil for processed foods.

Added Sugar Is Obesity's Best Friend, and it's Here to Stay

There's another important crop that's subsidized in the United States. Sugar cane.

Professor Barry Popkin says that added sugar is in 75% of food and drink that you'll find in today's grocery store. I shop at a massive organic food store that's supposed to be full of healthy food, and I am *extremely limited* if I want to avoid added sweetener products. Sugar and its variants are added to salad dressing, bread, ketchup, frozen meals, granola, cereal, and more. If you want a challenge, try to find cereal or granola without added sweetener. It's not easy. Better yet, try to find bread without added sweetener. That is surprisingly difficult.

If 75% of food in stores already contains added sugar, much of which is in the form of corn-derived, high-fructose corn syrup (HFCS), that means many billions of dollars are at stake, and powerful companies have a vested interest in protecting their sugar-based products, even if it means the demise of the health of modern society. No company will ever sacrifice themselves for humanity. That's not what for-profit companies are built to do.

Many of the world's societies are now trained to prefer sugary ultra-processed foods, and social dynamics are such that we care more about whether others are eating it than what the food will do to us. We also tend to assume that if everyone else is eating it, it must be fine. Unfortunately, "everyone else" has become overweight and disease prone! To be exact, 1.9 billion adults in 2014—almost one third of the entire world—were overweight. In the United States, almost 70% of people are overweight or obese. This has tipped the social influence scales in the wrong direction, because a society of overweight people will generally act the same way that made them overweight.

Look around you, and you'll see a general attitude of indulgence and near-worship of processed food. If one of my friends posts a picture of processed comfort food, the reactions are always positive. These foods have retained a remarkable amount of goodwill, considering the amount of damage they've caused to the human race.

If you follow the money, it's no wonder why processed food is so heavily marketed. If you follow the money, it's no wonder why soy, corn, and wheat are in so many foods. If you follow the money, it's no wonder why sugar is in 75% of all foods you'll find in a grocery store.

Business decisions are primarily driven by money. That's why food has become increasingly unhealthy but profitable. That's why we grow a disproportionate amount of certain crops. That's why obesity rates are rising and likely will continue to rise. This is not a conspiracy theory. It's plainly obvious that companies are loyal to their shareholders rather than the health of modern civilization. And let's not forget that humans enjoy these foods that harm our health.

We still have the ability to change. We can still choose the food we eat, and our choices will shape the future of food over time. The most important dietary choice you make is likely your consumption of added sweeteners. They're terrible for our weight and health, and they're in most food.

Sweeteners: Pick Your Poison, or Pick None

Refined sugar intake is associated with greater risk for obesity, gout, diabetes, and heart disease (to name a few).[62] It's even been associated with damage to the brain.[63] When sugar consumption is reduced, improvements to metabolic health are apparent,[64] which is important because obesity is primarily a metabolic problem. This is why reducing sugar intake is the frontline battle of weight loss (and why low-carb diets are generally most effective in the short term).

Half of Americans drink sugary drinks daily. They comprise about 10% of total calorie intake in the United States—[65]this is a *major* contributing cause of obesity. Did you know the serving size of sodas has more than tripled since the 1950s?

The Evolution of Soda Container Size (According to Harvard)[66]
Before the 1950s: 6.5 ounces
1960: 12 ounces
1990s: 20 ounces

Those are just the standard sizes. Movie and fast food cups today can be as large as 64 ounces (for soda, that is 192 grams of sugar). In the early 1980s, most soft drinks went through another unfortunate change—from being sweetened with sugar to high-fructose corn syrup. As bad as added sugar is for our health and weight, this lab creation appears to be even worse, especially when it comes to our weight.

High-Fructose Corn Syrup (HFCS)

Princeton researchers ran some experiments on rats with HFCS and sucrose. Here's what they found:

- "When rats are drinking high-fructose corn syrup at levels well below those in soda pop, they're becoming obese—every single one, across the board. Even when rats are fed a high-fat diet, you don't see this; they don't all gain extra weight."
- "The rats in the Princeton study became obese by drinking high-fructose corn syrup, but not by drinking sucrose."
- "In the 40 years since the introduction of high-fructose corn syrup as a cost-effective sweetener in the American diet, rates of obesity in the U.S. have skyrocketed, according to the Centers for Disease Control and Prevention. [...] High-fructose corn syrup is found in a wide range of foods and beverages, including fruit juice, soda, cereal, bread, yogurt, ketchup and mayonnaise. On average, Americans consume 60 pounds of the sweetener per person every year."
- "In contrast [to high fructose corn syrup], every fructose molecule in sucrose that comes from cane sugar or beet sugar is bound to a corresponding glucose molecule and must go through an extra metabolic step before it can be utilized."[67]

Our body has to work harder to break down natural foods for digestion. Think of it like internal exercise. It burns more calories, while giving our systems time to absorb the nutrients properly. Sugar is more easily absorbed than most food, but it is incrementally more challenging to absorb than high-fructose corn syrup.

Artificial Sweeteners

Artificial sweeteners are not the answer, either. Their impact on health is not fully understood, with some studies seeing no ill effects and others linking them to diseases as serious as cancer. If you only want to believe the ones that say they're safe, that's your choice. But you should know that their propensity to wreck our metabolism is more of a known quantity.

A study found that artificially sweetened beverages massively increased people's risk for type 2 diabetes (even more so than sugar-sweetened beverages).[68] The same effect was not seen in 100% fruit juice (mind you, fruit juice is still a weight-gaining drink). Another study found they were associated with an increased risk of metabolic syndrome.[69] And the most troubling of all was a study that found artificial sweeteners induced glucose intolerance by altering gut bacteria.[70] Yikes!

Why would artificially sweetened products cause metabolic problems? They seem to confuse our internal reward system. Food is rewarding biologically at two levels called sensory and postingestive. First, when pleasant-tasting food hits the tongue, our taste buds tell the brain, "Hey! Sweetness!", and we get a sensory reward. Then, after we ingest food, the metabolic and nutritive properties of the food provide us with a second reward of biological satisfaction.[71] This reward system helps us to regulate our food intake, because our desire for food rewards decreases after consumption (it's supposed to, anyway). Artificial sweeteners, however, provide a weaker initial reward than sugar at taste and almost completely bypass the postingestive reward system (because they're not food).

We trick the body when we consume artificial sweeteners, but not in the way we want. There's no way to trick your secondary reward system, which is based on the energy impact of food.

Drinking zero-calorie sweetened beverages seems too good to be true because it is. It's trying to get the pleasure from sweetness without the caloric consequences. It's a brilliant idea, honestly, but our bodies know it's not sugar when it can't be digested and used for energy. When we want something (sugar), and we're *teased* with the idea of it (zero calorie sweetener), we will only want it more.

In case you were curious, rats are the same way: "When a flavor was arbitrarily associated with high or low caloric content, rats ate more chow following a pre-meal with the flavor predictive of low caloric content.[72] These studies pose a hypothesis: Inconsistent coupling between sweet taste and caloric content can lead to compensatory overeating and positive energy balance."[73]

No Reward? No Deal

Artificial sweeteners are not rewarding biologically, and that's a problem. The concept of substitution is valuable for behavior change, but the new behavior needs *to offer a similar reward*, since rewards powerfully guide our behaviors. Artificial sweeteners work as a taste substitute for sugar and they are calorie free, but their weak activation of only one of the two food reward pathways is actually harmful for someone trying to reduce their intake of sweet foods.

"Lack of complete satisfaction, likely because of the failure to activate the postingestive component, further fuels the food seeking behavior. Reduction in reward response may contribute to obesity."[74]

Artificial sweeteners are not just a little bit sweeter than sugar; they are *hundreds of times* sweeter than sugar. Think about that. If something tastes *much* sweeter than sugar, it creates an even higher expectation for a significant reward. When it's finally processed, and provides you with almost no reward, what effect will that have? Disappointment and frustration. Even if you don't consciously feel that way, rest assured, your body will. When your body feels deprived of a reward, it will subtly (or not so subtly) find a way to get it later with cravings and "just this once" exceptions; it will use any trick it can to get you to indulge later.

By only partially activating the reward pathway (not to satisfaction), artificial sweeteners merely tease us. Teasing increases desire. "Artificial sweeteners, precisely because they are sweet, encourage sugar craving and sugar dependence. Repeated exposure trains flavor preference."[75]

That last sentence is crucial to everything in this book. Repeated exposure trains flavor preference.[76] Our food habits are not much different from any of our other habits. Those who frequently consume artificially sweetened goods are training themselves to be sugar addicts, and sugar addicts gain weight.

There was a nine-year observational study done on artificially sweetened beverage consumption and rates of overweight and obesity. Based on what we've discussed, can you guess what they found? "A significant positive dose-response relationship emerged between baseline ASB (artificially sweetened beverage) consumption and all outcome measures, adjusted for baseline BMI and demographic/behavioral characteristics."[77]

The outcome measures they speak of were overweight and obesity, meaning that those who consumed the most artificially sweetened beverages gained the most weight. To most, this result would seem a mystery, but you and I now know that those who consume artificial sweeteners tease themselves until indulgence.

Other Sweeteners
Stevia is probably healthier than artificial sweeteners, since it's naturally

derived. It is very sweet and very low calorie and appears to have fewer long-term health concerns than artificial sweeteners. The problem is that it too fails to activate the full reward pathway in the brain, which will cause the same issues as artificial sweeteners. This is a behavioral issue as much as it is a health issue—consuming sugar substitutes will *increase* your desire for sugar.

Sugar alcohols like xylitol, maltitol, sorbitol, and erythritol are lower in calories than sugar and contain similar sweetness. They are found naturally in some foods, but are often extracted and used in various processed foods. They are generally one of the best choices if you are adamant about using a sugar substitute, but beware, as they can cause gastrointestinal distress.

On Amazon, a 5-pound bag of Haribo gummy bears sweetened with maltitol received a number of hilarious reviews that went viral (if you need a hearty laugh, look no further than these reviews).[78] It appears some people underestimated the laxative power of maltitol and paid the price. One reviewer called it, "The Gummy Bear Cleanse." Be careful out there!

The best tolerated sugar alcohols are erythritol and xylitol, but you should know that xylitol is toxic to dogs.[79]

All in all, if you want something sweet, eat fruit first and real sugar second. Otherwise, you're taking a needless risk that could actually make you gain more weight. Additionally, real sugar doesn't give you the false sense of security that artificial sweeteners do.

In Defense of Fruit

If sugar is poor for our health but unprocessed foods are good for our health, where does that put fruit and unprocessed food relatively high in fructose?

The low-carbohydrate theory has made some people avoid fruit, and this is a big mistake. Many fruits and many vegetables are high in carbohydrates, and they've changed somewhat in the modern world because of selective breeding and agriscience, but not in a way that could possibly explain skyrocketing weight gain worldwide.

The studies I've seen on fruit are unanimous. Fruit is a weight-loss food. Anyone who says otherwise will cite two *theories*—the calorie content of fruit or the fructose/carb profile of fruit. These theories are not facts, especially because there is a lot of data—much of which I reference in this book—that debunks them.

A 2009 study of 77 overweight and obese people found that fruit consumption was associated with weight loss, not weight gain: "The relation between fruit consumption and body weight remained significant after controlling for age, gender, physical activity level, and daily macronutrient consumption. Further, increases in fruit consumption were associated with subsequent weight loss, controlling for the same covariates."[80] This says that fruit consumption created weight loss (which contradicts the fructose/carb theory), and that further increases in consumption lead to further weight loss (which contradicts the calorie theory). This is not theory; it's an observation of what happens when people eat fruit. But that was only 77 people, so let's look at some others.

The Verdict on Long-Term Fruit Consumption
Short-term thinking in the weight loss industry has placed too much weight (my puns are always intended) on short-term weight loss studies. Here are a couple of very long-term weight loss studies that deserve our attention.

In a 25-year study from 1986 to 2011 that included over 124,000 people, it was found that increased flavonoid consumption (primarily from fruit) led to weight loss, even "after adjustment for simultaneous changes in other lifestyle factors including other aspects of diet, smoking status, and physical activity."[81]

They found that the consumption of anthocyanins (a type of flavonoid) predicted the greatest weight loss. The main sources of anthocyanins in the study (and for most people who consume them) were blueberries and strawberries.

Flavonoid content might explain why people lose weight from increased fruit consumption. Studies on fructose look at its consumption in forms outside of fruit, such as in processed foods that contain high-fructose corn syrup. It's incorrect to then say that all foods with fructose are weight-gaining, just as it would be incorrect to assume that all foods with flavonoids are weight-reducing. If we added flavonoids to processed food, for example, the food would likely still be weight-gaining overall.

Harvard analyzed three cohort studies totaling more than 133,000 people over 24 years. They found that increased intake of non-starchy vegetables was associated with weight loss. Can you guess what was associated with even greater weight loss? Fruit consumption.[82]

Importantly, these associations are not guaranteed proof that fruit causes weight loss, as correlation is not causation. It's very likely to be the case, however, as fruit has so many weight loss-friendly features, dietary choices are known to cause weight gain or loss, and it is one of the "ancient" foods people ate long before the obesity crisis. The association of fruit consumption and weighing less is consistent across multiple long-term studies. Data like this is only surprising if you've been deceived into thinking that 100-calorie snack packs are the key to weight loss, or that "all carbs are fattening." Fruit has been demonized in many fad diets, yet it is consistently associated with the **most** weight loss among **all** food groups in long-term studies.

Seeing Is Believing

Imagine listening to someone lecture convincingly about why it's impossible for a hummingbird to fly. The lecturer explains in great scientific detail how the wings are too small to support the weight of its body. But just behind his head, you see a hummingbird flying. It's hovering in the same spot, flying backwards occasionally just to show off. Do you still believe the lecturer? The question we should be asking is not "Does fruit cause weight gain or weight loss?" Rather, we need to be asking "Why are we seeing that people lose weight as they eat more fruit?" The lecturer should do the same, and ask why he's seeing a hummingbird fly instead of lecturing others on why it shouldn't be able to fly.

To understand why a food relatively high in fructose isn't bad for our waistlines but good for them, we must look at the whole of fruit, not just its fructose content. What about its high water and fiber content? What about its bioavailable vitamins and minerals? What about its digestive enzymes? What about its superior anti-inflammatory effect compared to almost all foods, including many vegetables? What about the flavonoids? You can't forget the flavonoids! Calorie counters and anti-carbers suggest that these things don't matter because they've oversimplified food into macronutrient content. It may be simple to observe that people lose weight when eating fruit, but this simple and statistically relevant observation remains supreme in light of a food we don't completely understand. Here are a few reasons why fruit is a champion of weight loss.

1. Fruit tastes (really) good

This is not a joke. It's important! Fruit is a healthy and viable alternative for many of the sweet weight-gaining foods that people currently eat. Let's be real. You're not going to be able to replace your ice-cream gorging habit by stuffing your face with kale. But have you ever tasted mango? It's my favorite fruit. Its flavor and sweetness are completely satisfying. Have you ever eaten a frozen banana? It tastes like ice-cream. Try it.

Do you think it's coincidence that overweight people eat less fruit? "Overweight children (95th percentile) and obese adults (both genders) consumed significantly less fruit than healthy weight counterparts."[83] They're probably getting their sugar from processed foods.

Our tongues are equipped with taste buds to fully appreciate nature's sweetness. If we buy into the idea that fruit makes us fatter, despite science suggesting it makes us thinner, you can bet that we're going to seek out sweetness elsewhere (likely in the form of artificially sweetened or added-sugar processed foods, which actually do cause us to gain weight). Fruit is a vital outlet for your sweet tooth—when you crave something sweet, fruit is there to save the day!

2. Fruit contains enzymes, flavonoids, vitamins, and minerals

Fruit is one of the best sources for digestive enzymes. Proper digestion and assimilation of nutrients will reduce bloating and make you feel more satisfied and energetic. Two of my favorite fruits, pineapple and kiwifruit, contain potent enzymes called proteases that help you break down and digest protein. On a recent cruise, fresh pineapple was available at the buffet, and I ate it after every meal; I was amazed at the positive difference in my digestion and my complete lack of acid reflux for the entire trip.

Flavonoids appear to be underrated and not fully understood substances that make fruits several magnitudes healthier than their macronutrient profile makes them appear. Fruits are also loaded with bioavailable vitamins and minerals—our bodies need these micronutrients to function properly, and that includes weight management.

3. Unprocessed sugar in whole foods is better than chemicals, extractions, or added sugar

If you're aiming for a low-sugar diet, you might be tempted to skip fruit. Unless you medically can't have it, don't skip it. Fruit tends to be lower in sugar compared to processed foods. A 20-ounce soda contains more sugar than one banana, one apple, one orange, and one kiwi combined.

As for artificial sweeteners, they have zero calories because they aren't food. Cannonballs are zero calories and very filling. Why not eat one of those? Both added sugar and artificial sweeteners increase your risk for type 2 diabetes.[84] Shouldn't you at least avoid fruit just to lower your chance for diabetes? Of course not! A study found that "greater consumption of specific whole fruits, particularly blueberries, grapes, and apples, is significantly associated with a lower risk of type 2 diabetes, whereas greater consumption of fruit juice is associated with a higher risk."[85]

4. Fruit is sweet, but it still lowers blood sugar

It's counterintuitive that a food high in fructose could possibly lower blood sugar, but again, let's look at the data, not the theories. A study done in Mexico tested a low-fructose diet (less than 20g daily) against a moderate natural-fructose diet (50-70g daily). Both groups saw improvements to blood sugar, insulin resistance, cholesterol, and blood pressure. The biggest difference between the two groups was weight loss, as the natural-fructose group lost 50% more weight (4.2kg compared to 2.8kg). Cutting out all or most fructose in your diet will bring you some results; they just won't be as great if you also remove fruit.

5. Fruit has a fantastic satiety-to-calorie ratio

Remember when I told you I ate an entire bag of frozen mangoes? That 10-ounce (284g) bag of frozen sliced mangoes was only 200 calories, while a 52.7g Snicker's bar is 250 calories. The mangoes take up five times as much space in your stomach and provide far more micronutrients despite having fewer calories.

Our bodies are about 60-70% water.[86] In a way, eating more fruit is like drinking more water. In addition to its high water content, fruit is high in fiber, making it a very satiating food for relatively few calories.

WARNING: Fruit juice is not the same as whole fruit!

Fruit juice may contain some of the vitamins and minerals as the fruit it comes from, but it lacks the satiety that whole fruit provides. Whole fruit consumed before meals reduced caloric intake (of lunch) by 15% in a study. That's fantastic, but, interestingly enough, they found that "adding naturally occurring levels of fiber to [fruit] juice did not enhance satiety."[87] Even when you add the fiber back, fruit juice doesn't measure up to the natural satiety of whole fruit. (Apple sauce didn't have the same satiety effect either.)

Whole fruit regulates how much you eat and how your body absorbs the fructose. Fruit juice, even 100% fruit juice, makes you gain weight. It makes sense when you think about it. Studies find that fructose is weight-gaining, and squeezing the juice out of fruit isolates the fructose and loses everything contained in the pulp. The better alternative to fruit juice is fruit-infused water, which we'll talk about in the application chapter.

How Healthy Is Your Diet?

Now that we've discussed what sorts of foods are good and bad for weight loss, it's time to take a look at your current dietary habits. Some people are under the impression that they have already tried the "eat healthy foods" plan and failed, when in reality they've never tried. If your idea of healthy eating is off the mark, you'll gain weight, as you think you're doing the right thing.

"Healthy food" is far narrower than most people believe it to be. Healthy weight loss foods do NOT include things like low-fat flavored yogurt, organic granola bars, sugar-free anything, organic tortilla chips, organic candy, low-calorie diet foods, 100% fruit juice, organic or conventional processed foods, basically *anything* with added sugar (which is 75% of food in grocery stores), or salads drenched in high-fructose corn syrup and soybean oil dressing.

Here's the concerning data: In a *Consumer Reports* survey of 1,234 people, 89.7% of American respondents thought they consumed a diet that's at least "somewhat healthy."[88] And yet, 43% of these same people reported consuming at least one soda, Frappuccino, or bubble tea per day. If you consume any of those once per day, you almost certainly don't have a "somewhat healthy" diet.

Someone can drink one soda a day and think they're being healthy just because they have a friend who drinks three per day. Tell your pancreas not to worry about all the insulin it's pumping out, because Jimmy's pancreas has to do it three times a day. Or, in the case of artificial sweeteners, tell your dopaminergic pathways not to be too upset at the lack of reward, because Jimmy's reward system is even more screwed up.

Look in your kitchen. Are your counter and fridge/freezer stocked with fresh or frozen fruits and vegetables? If not, are they usually? If not, you probably don't have a healthy diet.

If almost 90% of Americans believe they eat a healthy diet, then we've got a serious denial problem. The aforementioned nationally representative cross-sectional study in the United States published in March 2016 found that "ultra-processed foods comprised 57.9% of total energy intake."[89] These are foods that would ideally comprise 0% of a human diet, and yet they're consumed the most.

Healthy Food Tiers

The (un)healthiness of food is almost completely based on how processed it is. Generally speaking, the more processed a food is, the more calorie dense, the less nutritional value, and the less satiating per calorie it is. There are nuances about which unprocessed foods are *best* for weight loss, but your progress won't be made or lost by eating peaches instead of grapes. It will be made or lost by how much real food you eat compared to how much processed food you eat. Processed food creates weight gain. Minimally processed food greatly assists with weight loss if you're overweight, or it can maintain your healthy weight if you aren't.

Dead Food
A plant leaf contains compounds such as chlorophyll and antioxidants that keep it healthy and alive. When you eat the plant, these living compounds are still active, and they will have similar life-promoting effects inside of your body. Have you ever tried to save an avocado for later and saw that it turned brown soon after? That's oxidation. Oxidation kills and impairs cellular function. Fat oxidation is the term for fat cells being destroyed for energy. Oxidation is good for fat, but not for most of the other cells in our body!

Processed food is dead. Processing kills the most beneficial parts of food.

For example, cereal is seen by many as "healthy" because it has a long list of added vitamins, but it has *almost none* of the beneficial compounds of a living food.

The Food Scale

With the exception of vegetables, people argue about how basically every other food affects weight. It's useful to know when to look at the big picture and when to look at the details, and this is a case where we need to look at the big picture. Worldwide obesity rates have climbed rapidly as we've created and consumed food from the lab more than from the farm. When ultra-processed food consumption spiked, calorie consumption spiked, and obesity rates spiked.

Most weight loss authors believe they have to come up with a definitive stance on every food, but this is totally unnecessary for weight loss. If you get the basics right, eat simple and real food, and stop eating large amounts of the obvious weight-gaining foods, you'll succeed.

Don't worry about eating or not eating debatable foods like potatoes, meat, whole wheat, and dairy. These foods have been eaten for centuries without associated weight problems. It's possible that any of these foods *may* tilt the scales in the wrong direction ever so slightly, but eating cooked potatoes will not *ruin* your weight loss efforts the way that frequent soda or croissant consumption will. Once you've established a clear pattern of eating healthy foods, then perhaps you can nitpick about things like dairy or whole grain bread. Dieting culture makes people worry about whole grain bread when they eat fast food every day. When you're eating mostly fresh fruits and vegetables, you've mastered the basics of healthy eating. Then you can move on to whether or not you should eat debatable foods. Until that happens, your job is to pursue good foods and not worry about *anything else you eat*. It bears repeating that the correct perspective to obtain a healthy diet is toward healthy food, not away from unhealthy food.

Please don't use the following list for dieting. This is just to give you an idea of where foods stand on the weight loss spectrum. It's important to know what foods are weight loss-friendly, but it's more important not to (try to) change your diet all at once. This list is not comprehensive. Try to understand the concepts underlying these foods.

1. Super-Healthy Foods: Weight Loss-Friendly as a Staple

After you read the others, come back up and read this list again, because this is the list that matters. It's not about what to avoid, it's about what to pursue. This seems like a short list until you consider that it says ALL fruits and (basically) ALL vegetables. There are 4,000 varieties of tomato, and that's just one fruit. There are thousands upon thousands of fruits and vegetables with different tastes, textures, and uses.

Generally speaking, if you eat a minimally processed fruit or vegetable, it will not contain a harmful amount of salt, sugar, calories, or fat. Avocados, for example, are 82% fat, but they are not obesogenic and offer terrific satiety: "A randomized single blinded, crossover postprandial study of 26 healthy overweight adults suggested that one-half an avocado consumed at lunch significantly reduced self-reported hunger and desire to eat, and increased satiation as compared to the control meal."[90]

- Water (This is one of the most underrated weight loss tools. We'll talk about this later.)
- All fruits
- (Almost) all vegetables
- Seeds, beans, and nuts
- Fish (not fried)
- Mustard
- Vinegar
- Eggs
- All spices
- All herbs (Spices and herbs make food delicious *and* they're good for you. It's almost unfair.)
- Fermented foods such as (full-fat) yogurt, kimchi, sauerkraut, kefir, komboucha, etc.
- Olive oil
- Coconut oil

Coconut oil is excellent for weight loss as it's very high in medium chain triglycerides (MCTs), which are quickly absorbed and used for energy (rather than stored as fat). There's no need to cook with anything else besides coconut oil, olive oil, or butter. Coconut oil and olive oil are versatile, delicious, and healthy. Olive oil is also great for cold uses like dip or dressing.

In a clever "real world" experiment, Professor Grootveld analyzed leftover oils after volunteers had cooked with them. He found that "sunflower oil and corn oil produced aldehydes at levels 20 times higher than recommended by the World Health Organization. Olive oil and rapeseed oil produced far fewer aldehydes, as did butter and goose fat."[91] Aldehydes are oxidized alcohols that are toxic to us and linked to many diseases. Among all oils, coconut oil produces the least amount of aldehydes when heated for cooking.[92]

Note: Green (vegetable-only) juices and smoothies are nutrition powerhouses. They are a good addition to one's diet for their anti-inflammatory and nutrient-absorption benefits. The key word there is addition. Don't starve yourself and force green juice down your throat. That's trendy, but not sustainable.

2. Moderately Healthy Foods: Weight Loss-Friendly in Moderation

Whole grains: Grains such as brown rice, whole wheat pasta, quinoa, barley, millet, oats, and so on are healthy (this doesn't include crackers or most breads, which generally contain multiple processed ingredients).

Minimally processed meat: I know. It's popular these days to blame meat, but we've been omnivores a very long time without weight problems. Plus, I think it's difficult to sustain yourself on a vegetarian or vegan diet. That said, if you prefer eating vegetarian or vegan, you could do much worse!

3. Debatable Foods

Many whole grain breads contain additional ingredients, so if you're going to pick one go-to source for wheat, choose whole grain pasta (one ingredient). Some people have an allergy to wheat, but if that's you, you don't need me to tell you not to eat it. Since pasta sauce almost always contains added sugar, I like to use olive oil, pesto, and cheese for flavor. It's healthy and delicious! You can also make your own pasta sauce pretty easily.

Full-fat dairy: Dairy is a high-calorie category of food, but its calories are high-quality and satiating. One study found that while on a calorie restriction diet, those who included dairy in their diet lost 70% more weight (and those who included calcium lost 26% more weight).[93] If you enjoy dairy, consume it moderately, but still aim for the super-healthy foods as your go-to staples, and you'll do well.

Whether to consume full-fat or non-fat dairy is not debatable. For milk, sour cream, butter, or yogurt, and other dairy foods, go full-fat.

- In one study, the BMI was lower in women who consumed more whole-fat dairy products.[94] A study of over 18,000 women found that "greater intake of high-fat dairy products, but not intake of low-fat dairy products, was associated with less weight gain."[95]
- A study of over 1,700 men came to the exact same conclusion. Full-fat dairy decreased odds of obesity 12 years later, and low-fat dairy was associated with increased rates of obesity.[96]
- A study of children from 2 to 4 years old found that those who drank 1% or skim milk had the highest body mass index compared to those who drank 2% or whole milk.[97]

I couldn't find any studies that found low-fat milk to be superior to whole milk in any way, probably because it's worse in *every way*. Oregon State Agricultural College published a bulletin in 1930 titled "Fattening Pigs for Market." Take a look at this interesting quote I plucked from the bulletin: "Skim milk. This is not only the very best supplement for growing pigs, but is of almost equal value for fattening purposes."[98] It seems that, in many ways, our knowledge of weight management has regressed. We used to correctly feed pigs skim milk to fatten them, and now we drink it ourselves as a "weight loss drink."

Such data makes complete sense in light of everything we've discussed, and it surprises calorie counters and "fat is bad" pitchforkers, who base their conclusions on ONE facet of complex foods. Read the following sentence, look at the studies again, and internalize what this means: **Full-fat milk contains almost double the calories of non-fat milk for the same serving size.**

Are you going to trust the prevailing theories (that have allowed obesity to skyrocket)? Or will you consider what theories best explain observational science? Here's an explanation about dairy that actually fits the data, which clearly says full-fat milk is better than non-fat milk for weight loss: Whole milk is less tampered with, a whole and natural food. Skim milk is a *more processed version* of whole milk. While that's not a particularly strong argument, since it requires you to first accept the "processed is worse" idea, this is: If you drink skim milk, you will be less satiated and satisfied than if you drink whole milk. You will likely be less satiated *per calorie* with non-fat or low-fat milk. Four ounces of whole milk could be more satisfying and filling than 8 ounces of skim milk. If we put milk consumption in a vacuum, then, sure, skim milk has fewer calories and would mean less weight gain. But the food we eat now affects the type and quantity of food we'll eat later. In addition, the fat in milk slows the digestion of its sugars.

Your body is not going to think, "Oh, it's the same amount of milk, but half the calories!" Skim milk only fools the person who drinks it (not their body). *The human body cannot be tricked into weight loss.* Enjoy your dairy as full fat if you want to lose weight. You don't have to take my word for it or buy my proposed theories on milk. Just look at the data. Of course, raw milk is far better than store-bought milk because it's not processed with pasteurization (heated to high temperatures to kill everything) and homogenization (spun rapidly to remove cream separation). Raw milk is alive. It contains beneficial enzymes that are otherwise destroyed in pasteurization, but it's not always easy to access. It's actually illegal in the USA to sell raw milk for personal consumption. "Pets" can drink it though. Raw milk has some risk for bacterial contamination such as salmonella and listeria, so consume it at your own risk.

Protein powder: If you're going to have protein shakes, it's best to have them in the morning for breakfast, and it's best to get some with limited added ingredients (I use Promix and Solgar). I prefer whey protein over others for its complete protein profile. It is a processed food, but it's one of the better ones if you choose one with the right ingredients. Protein is highly satiating and great for building or maintaining muscle mass. As such, a good protein powder can be helpful for redistributing weight from fat to muscle, especially if you're exercising. What's better than a protein shake in the morning? Whole fruits, vegetables, eggs, minimally processed meat, or yogurt.

Soup: It's usually a good choice (high water content), but it greatly depends on how it's made and what it contains!

Super-starchy vegetables: Potatoes, peas, and corn are only listed here because they were associated with weight gain in the 24-year study mentioned earlier. Potatoes in particular are demonized by many, but they look great on paper. They're the world's most satiating food, and they are packed with antioxidants, vitamins, and minerals. Potatoes have been a staple food in many countries throughout history. Obesity and overweight to the present extent are a modern phenomenon with a modern cause. That's not to say that you won't gain some weight if you stuff yourself with potatoes—the research is mixed—but it does mean you can eat potatoes without worry. If you love potatoes, as many do, you could do much worse.

White rice: It's not the worst food you can eat and it's leagues better than ultra-processed food. Additionally, many cultures have stayed thin and healthy on a diet heavy in white rice. That said, if you can switch to brown rice, do it! White rice is processed to eliminate the germ and bran of brown rice, which means you get less fiber and (far) fewer nutrients. If you have to choose between white rice and white bread, white rice wins in a landslide because white bread is processed to an extreme (often with *dozens* of ingredients). White rice is just a one-ingredient food, which is a big plus. That being said, if you get white rice in a restaurant, don't count on it being only one ingredient. It's often cooked with oil and added sodium.

4. Semi-Unhealthy Foods: Might Cause Weight Gain
Low-fat or no-fat dairy: Beneficial fats are taken out, making it less satiating than full-fat dairy, and unlike full-fat dairy, it's also mostly associated with weight gain in studies. Remember, they used skim milk in the 1930s to fatten pigs.

Fruit smoothies: If you get a fruit smoothie at a chain, it will almost definitely contain added sugar and/or consist of fruit-flavored syrup instead of actual fruit. Even if you make the smoothie at home with real fruit, you're missing out on the true fiber content of the fruit, as studies have found that blending the fruit changes how the fiber is digested. This makes it closer to fruit juice, which is a definite weight-gaining drink!

5. Super-Unhealthy Foods: Weight-Gaining
Ultra-processed foods: chips, crackers, cookies, pies, cakes, ice-cream, pancakes, waffles, white pasta, pizza, white bread, fruit juice (yes, even 100% juice), soda, lattes, and candy. If reading that list made you salivate, don't worry, because healthy food can make you salivate too!

Anything fried, and most things cooked in vegetable oil: Soybean oil and most other vegetable oils are big contributors to weight gain and they are *extremely* difficult to avoid in the United States.

Faux healthy foods: These include organic granola bars (added sugar), organic dried fruit (usually has added sugar and it's missing important water content), flavored yogurt (always has added sweetener), organic cereal (highly processed with added sugar).

Most commonly available sauces and dressings: Since most sauces are high in soybean oil, sugar, and/or salt, they're big weight-gainers. Almost every commercial salad dressing I've seen uses soybean oil.

Significantly processed meat: Meats like bologna, hot dogs, and so on are processed to the point that it becomes challenging to still call them "meat."

Side note: I avoid canned food, because most cans contain the synthetic compound known as BPA, which is not only associated with obesity[99] but also insulin resistance[100] and cancer.[101] Dr. Ana Soto said, "If we take the results in animal models together, I think we have enough evidence to conclude that BPA increases the risk for breast and prostate cancer in humans."[102] The BPA in can liners does leach into the food. A Harvard study found that daily canned soup consumption raised participants' urine levels of BPA by 1,221% compared to those who ate fresh soup.[103] You can't argue with that. Thankfully, more companies are moving to BPA-free cans. I recommend fresh food, frozen food, glass jar food, or if cans are a must, try to find BPA-free canned food. If canned food is the only way you'll eat vegetables and you don't have access to BPA-free canned food, I think it's still worth it to eat vegetables in whatever way you can.

Healthy Drinking
One of the most effective weight loss methods is so obvious we all missed it. Drink water! It is zero calories and helps regulate appetite (diet drinks are zero calories too, but they hurt your metabolism as water improves it).

If you habitually drink anything but water, be suspicious of what it does to your waistline. Soda, fruit juice, alcohol, and any other drink with added sugar (including coffee and tea) work against your goal to lose fat. Milk is a question mark.

A study divided 48 people into two groups. Both groups consumed a low-calorie diet, but one group drank two 8-ounce cups of water before meals. At the end of 12 weeks, the water-drinking group lost 15.5 pounds, compared to the other group's 11 pounds.[104] The folly of calorie restriction and the short duration of the study aside, the water-drinking group was the clear winner. Calorie restriction diets cause our bodies to try to store more fat in the long term, but drinking more water might just do the opposite. A study of seven men and seven women found that drinking 500 ml of water (16.9 oz bottle) increased their metabolic rate by 30% in 40 minutes.[105] Increased metabolism is a very good sign, even if it's only observed in the short term. The key issue with low-calorie diets is that metabolism plummets. Even if a food made people gain weight in the short term, but increased their metabolism in the long term, it would still be excellent for weight loss, and *far superior* to methodologies that bring short-term weight loss and long-term metabolic devastation and weight gain. This is theoretical discussion, of course, as drinking water helps our health and weight management now and later.

There is one other special drink that deserves mentioning. Other than water, green tea could be argued as the ultimate weight loss drink for its unique antioxidant content. Studies show green tea specifically helps burn visceral fat in the abdominal area.[106] This is the area where people generally prefer to lose fat, and it's also the most harmful fat on the body. Green tea's fat-burning effect is largely due to high amounts of an antioxidant called catechin. From my research, this antioxidant is also found in other foods like cocoa, blackberries, and red wine, but green tea has the highest amount of catechins of any food.

What about coffee and tea? Caffeine can be beneficial in small doses for raising metabolism temporarily. In fact, as one of the most common ingredients in pre-workout supplements, caffeine is probably best used to enhance your workout. Of course, if you "need" caffeine to have energy, then that's not ideal. I don't drink coffee, because I've seen too many people become dependent on it for energy.

In regards to health and weight, the biggest issue with coffee and tea is the added sweeteners. If you have to choose one, honey, raw brown sugar, and stevia appear to be the lesser of the evils (I would choose honey). One thing is for certain—regular coffee and tea are much better than sugary lattes and other "signature" drinks at coffee shops. If it's between a cup of coffee and a caramel latte, the coffee wins in a landslide.

I can tell you one thing: If you're able to disassociate drinking beverages and sweetness, you're way ahead of the game. This all comes down to conditioning. To the person who drinks soda daily, water tastes bland. To the person who drinks water daily, sodas and lattes taste too sweet.

Liquids satisfy our thirst, and there is inherent satisfaction in that. The base of all drinks is water, which means that drinking water can become a habit and beverage that you enjoy, even if you're not particularly fond of it now. We can learn to enjoy the things that satisfy our needs.

Alcohol

When it comes to alcohol, wine is the winner for health and weight loss. Regular wine consumption is associated with lower mortality than in non-drinkers and drinkers of other alcohol types.[107] Its intake has a "J-shaped" relationship with death—it's a healthy drink in moderation that becomes unhealthy if you overindulge.

There's no hard evidence that wine or alcohol of any kind is a "weight loss drink." A 13-year Harvard study with 19,200 women found that those who consumed alcohol gained less weight than non-drinkers, but they still gained weight (red wine had the best inverse association with overweight and obesity).[108]

Red wine does contain the antioxidant resveratrol, which has been shown to be excellent for both health and weight management. But you can get this antioxidant in much higher quantities from eating fruits like blueberries, grapes, strawberries, raspberries, and apples.[109] For alcohol, the best choice is red wine (drink it by the glass, not the bottle).

Exercise Matters, But Not for the Reason You Think

We've talked a lot about food, but what about exercise? Does it really help us lose weight?

The books that tell you exercise isn't necessary for weight loss make four mistakes.

1. They fail to consider the long-term positive metabolic effect of consistent exercise (by only looking at short-term studies on exercise and weight loss).
2. They assume that diet and exercise together are "too much" for the person to handle, and thus, bank heavily on the more important half (diet); it's only too much if your strategy is dieting.
3. They don't mention the difference between exercising and being active.
4. They fail to consider the value of exercise as stress relief to reduce emotional eating, lower cortisol levels, and

improve sleep.

The weight loss effect of exercising has ironically become a debated point. Short-term studies show that most diets work and exercise doesn't help with weight loss, but long-term studies show that most diets *don't work* and that exercise is one of the key factors in successful and lasting weight loss. So we have a choice—do we emphasize short-term studies or long-term studies? Long-term studies show real, lasting change. Short-term studies might show that the "The Gummy Bear Cleanse" is the most effective weight loss method. One reviewer claimed to lose four pounds in only one day. Now that's a result!

If you base your conclusions on short-term studies of a year or less, you're going to favor short-term strategies that almost always fail in the long term. Why is anyone surprised when a 10-day weight loss plan doesn't bring *lasting* results? It's 10 days! Like a submarine's inability to fly, it's not designed for that.

Exercise Is Not About "Burning Calories"

Short-term studies show that exercise is an ineffective method of weight loss.[110] This is partly true, in that the amount of *calories* you burn exercising will have, at best, a slight impact on your weight in the near future. Also, when you exercise, your appetite typically increases, which leads to eating more food, making the total caloric deficit less significant than one might think. But again, this is narrow-mindedly looking at calories only. There's more at play here, and the science shows that.

A meta-analysis found that "Weight loss is similar in the short term for diet-only and combined BWMPs (behavioral weight management programs) but in the longer term weight loss is increased when diet and physical activity are combined."[111] The National Weight Control Registry studies people who have achieved lasting weight loss. They say of members who lose weight and keep it off for years, "90% exercise, on average, about 1 hour per day."[112]

Let's look *really* long-term on this one. A 20-year study found that exercise was associated with decreased weight gain and a smaller waist in men and (especially) women.[113] How exercise specifically improves long-term weight loss isn't 100% understood, but it's been shown to help. A good guess? Obesity is basically a body out of balance, and exercise improves nearly every bodily function, so it may help to rebalance how the body intakes and uses energy (metabolism).

There's some evidence that exercise aids weight loss by optimizing your body's hormones. Studies have found that regular exercise is associated with lower insulin resistance and higher insulin sensitivity in people (both of which are positive metabolic attributes for health and weight).[114]

Fat Loss Beats Weight Loss

Even if you aren't losing *weight* while exercising, you still could be losing *fat*. "The findings from four nonrandomized or controlled studies report that exercise with or without weight loss is associated with reductions in both visceral and subcutaneous fat."[115] This is critical, because reduction in fat is the true goal, and if you stay at the same weight but have traded fat for increased muscle, you're going to look and feel better.

Exercise is not about "burning calories." It's about the metabolic, anti-inflammatory, and circulatory benefits. When you view it as such, quotes like this one from a study will no longer scare you: "To our surprise, we have found that exercise has little, if any, effect on 24-hour fat oxidation."[116] Exercise is a healthy lifestyle choice, not a short-term weight loss miracle. By exercising, you will see weight loss results in the long term in addition to numerous health benefits.

If you don't currently exercise, that probably means you don't enjoy doing it. I'm aware of that and that's okay, because mini habits can change that preference. One push-up a day changed my lazy self from resisting exercise to enjoying it and doing it several times per week. Anyone can do it.

Exercise is not a sacrifice you make to lose weight; it's one of the most enjoyable parts of life that many people haven't been able to enjoy. When you're out of shape, it's not much fun and feels uncomfortable to exercise, but once you start experiencing the benefits and getting stronger, you'll get hooked. With this book, you have the best strategy to get to that point.

Hidden Weight Loss Factors

Food and movement are the primary two factors associated with weight loss discussion, but a few other factors deserve consideration, too. These factors can directly or indirectly affect weight by changing the way we move and eat.

Sleep

A study of ten people found that a lack of sleep sabotaged weight loss. It slowed fat loss by 55%, increased non-fat loss by 60%, and shifted hormones to favor increased hunger and decreased fat oxidation. This was the result of 5.5 hours of sleep compared to 8.5 hours of sleep.[117] This study was interesting, because they tested each person twice for two weeks at 5.5 hours of sleep and then for two weeks at 8.5 hours of sleep. These differences were observed in the same people, and because they controlled participants' calorie intake, the differences were minimized. When the people slept less, they were hungrier, which would make them susceptible to overeating. With even energy intake, their fat loss was hindered on less sleep.[118]

A larger study of 1,024 people found that shorter sleep resulted in lower leptin, higher ghrelin (the hunger hormone), and increased body mass index. Below the eight-hour mark, "increased BMI was proportional to decreased sleep."[119]

To support the findings of these studies, what's your experience been? Have you noticed that you tend to eat more when sleep deprived? I do. I remember some days of sleep deprivation in which my stomach seemed to be a bottomless pit of hunger.

Being that the key to lasting change is to make success easier than failure, not getting enough sleep is a *serious* hindrance to weight loss. It puts you at a severe biological disadvantage compared to getting enough sleep (of which the consensus is 7-9 hours).

Stress Levels

Cortisol is the hormone released when we're stressed, and too much of it causes the body to store fat in the abdominal area. That's not what we want, so the answer is to destress. That's easier said than done, but it's also easier to do than one might think. If you actively try to reduce stress in your life, you can succeed, but very few people plan ways to destress. Some of my favorite ways to relax are meditation, massages, playing basketball, and using sensory deprivation tanks.

Fun

"Across three studies, in both lab and field settings, we found that framing a physical activity as fun (vs. exercise) influenced participants' subsequent behavior. Specifically, we found that labeling a physical activity as fun reduced the amount of calories consumed in side dishes during a meal (study 1), the amount of hedonic food served (study 2), and perception of fun during a race positively influenced the choice of a healthy snack (study 3)."[120] If you perceive your weight loss journey as "work," you're missing out on the advantages of a fun perspective.

Simultaneous Change
You're better off changing your diet and exercise at the same time, as diet and exercise can form a virtuous cycle together. A study of 200 people found that simultaneous change of diet and exercise improved adherence compared to starting one and adding the other later.[121]

Gut Health
Gut health is a growing field of science, including how it relates to weight loss. Scientists have found differences in the gut bacteria of overweight people (and rats) compared to their healthy weight counterparts. Fermented foods (e.g., yogurt, sauerkraut, kefir, kimchi, komboucha) are so healthy because they repopulate the stomach with beneficial bacteria.

While these fringe factors might not seem important, they can make a big difference, so keep them in mind.

Side Benefits of Mini Habits
Mini habits directly improve three of these hidden factors. First, they're fun. They're more fun than any other weight loss plan you've tried before. This strategy doesn't ban you from eating any foods; it's rooted in positivity and daily success, and it delivers outsized results compared to how easy the behaviors are. Compared to dieting, mini habits are like a theme park.

Mini habits also allow you to change your exercise and eating habits simultaneously without burning out. With traditional change methods, even two synergistic changes like this are extremely difficult to sustain. Since you can maintain several mini habits at a time, you'll be able to make progress in both of these areas simultaneously and benefit from their synergy.

Finally, mini habits can decrease your stress levels. When you are less demanding of yourself and still get results, life feels easier and more relaxed. This can then improve your sleep.

If You Think I'm Wrong...

I've presented my case for how weight gain and weight loss work.

After looking at hundreds of studies and analyzing their data, the only consistent finding was that processed foods cause weight gain, not carbs or fat or calories. We've had all of those other things for as long as we've existed, and the underlying, core theory behind each of these weight loss theories is that now we eat too much of them. They say we eat too many carbs, too much fat, or too many calories.

The modern Western diet is now measurably higher in ultra-processed foods than it is in real food,[122] **and that is why 70% of Americans are overweight. Other countries who have followed suit have become more obese.**

If you happen to disagree with me, that's fine, because this is only the second biggest problem of the weight loss industry. The *biggest* problem is not with nutrition-based diets, which generally promote healthier eating: it's with the way people are taught to implement them. *Mini Habits for Weight Loss* isn't a new diet, it's a new *approach* to weight loss. If you have a particular diet or way of eating that you believe is best for your long-term interests, you can adapt these principles to implement it more effectively.

Part Two

Introduction: Strategy Rules

Welcome to part two, my favorite part of the book. Part one discussed the keys to successful weight loss; part two converts what we've learned from part one into an actionable strategy that works. The next three chapters are general strategy, food strategy, and fitness strategy.

In the upcoming chapter, we'll talk about our general weight loss strategy. That is, how are we going to think about our big picture attempt to lose weight? Is it ideal to think of yourself as "trying to lose weight" or is it better to aim to maintain your weight instead?

The food strategy chapter is next, and it addresses how to think about food. It will answer questions like, "Should I ban junk food?" and "When will I know to stop eating?" and "What if I don't like vegetables?"

After that, we'll discuss fitness strategy and answer questions such as, "What's the best form of exercise for weight loss?" and "How much should I exercise?" and "Does chasing my kids around the house count as exercise?"

"Where Are the Mini Habits?"

Since weight loss encompasses your entire lifestyle, there are factors to consider beyond what daily mini habits you choose to do. Strategy has two components—how we think about something, and what we physically do. There are a number of important psychological dispositions that can make or break your attempts. We'll cover those and discuss the advantages of mini habits before closing out the food and fitness chapters with specific mini habit ideas.

Practicing your mini habits will gradually change the way you think, but you'll be even more likely to succeed if you have the right perspective to go along with your mini habits.

5
General Strategy

Look, If it Were Intuitive, We'd All Be Slender Billionaires[123]

"For changes to be of any true value, they've got to be lasting and consistent."
~ Tony Robbins

The Benefits of the Hard Path

Exercise and healthy eating are the hard path. Exercise makes almost all internal bodily processes and functions more efficient: it improves insulin function to better energize cells, increases blood flow to more easily disperse nutrients, and optimizes hormone levels. Good, real food provides micronutrients and unique compounds to improve organ function and reduce inflammation.

Aside from those "concrete benefits" of healthy living, you will also become stronger by taking the hard path. If you climb a mountain every day, a walk up the staircase is easy. But if you drive your car between sitting sessions all day, a walk up the staircase can be grueling. It's beneficial for us to take the harder route because it makes *everything else* easier. Humans are smart, and we recognize this, but many people fail to consider their willpower limitations and overwhelming preference to take the easy path. We often succumb to the easy path, even when trying to take the harder, more beneficial path. The hard path is only beneficial if you actually take it! But how can we take it consistently?

Every other book will tell you to grit your teeth and just do it, or, even worse, they'll tell you that you need to "want it more." Basically, they'll tell you to throw everything you have at your goal. Do whatever it takes to take the hard path, eat your vegetables, and get to the gym. If you fail, it's your fault. How stupid. The smartest strategy harmonizes our natural preference (the easy path) with our unique power of choice.

If you need to take the hard path, but you like the easy path, you must make the harder path easier, and the easier path harder. Do you see now why mini habits are a powerful strategy? Mini habits make it easy to take life's most difficult (and beneficial) paths.

The Importance of Perceived Difficulty
Doing 30 minutes of moderate intensity exercise on an exercise bike requires a certain amount of effort, and you can't change that. You can, however, change your likelihood of getting on the bike through strategy, which can change your perspective, and your perspective changes the *perceived difficulty* of a task.

Imagine that Jim and Sam are people of equal ability who attempt the same challenge. Their ability and task difficulty are objectively identical, but Sam thinks the challenge is fun and Jim thinks the challenge is boring. Who do you think will find the challenge easier? Sam will, because he thinks it's fun. Your perspective is powerful enough to make a difficult task easy or an easy task difficult.

A mini habit in practice changes your relationship with a behavior over time by creating a new expectation. Practicing piano is naturally harder to do than watching television, so a mini habit makes it comparably easy by asking you to play one song a day, or even to sit down at the piano and open your songbook. Exercising is harder than reading the newspaper, so a mini habit makes it comparably easy by asking you to do just one push-up (and more only if you so choose). Eating broccoli is harder than eating cake, so a mini habit makes it comparably easy by asking you to eat one piece of broccoli.

By making the hard path easier to take, you destroy the very foundation of what sustains unhealthy behavior and keeps healthy behavior a "someday" dream. Unhealthy behavior is so common not just because it's easy, but because societies make it *seem easy*. Healthy behavior is actually not much more challenging than unhealthy behavior, but it becomes so when framed that way.

Why is it that a person will sit down to watch a one-minute YouTube video without thinking about it, but not run in place for one minute because "it's not a full workout?" It's okay to sit for a minute, but not good enough to exercise for the same amount of time? That's why people sit for eight hours a day and don't exercise very much. Why is it that eating salad is a special dietary decision, while eating a burger is normal? This needs to be reversed! The rare, special behaviors we put on a pedestal are the least likely ones to impact our lives. Your mini habits will transform these "special healthy behaviors" into normal ones that have a chance to become habits and change your life.

This is the framework of thinking behind the *Mini Habits* strategy. You'll set easy, doable daily mini habits to form habits in high impact areas. Since we're focused on weight loss and that entails many non-habitual choices too, you'll also learn to make non-habitual healthy choices into some of the easiest, most casual choices you can make.

Nobody blames a sprinter for running in a straight line toward the finish line, because that's the fastest and easiest way to cover the distance. Nobody scolds a basketball player for dunking the ball, when he could step back and try a more difficult fade away jumper. The easy path is always smarter, except when there are derivative consequences (like gaining weight) or when the hard path has derivative benefits worth pursuing (such as lifting weights to get stronger).

Sitting down all day is easier than standing, but it's associated with mortality and metabolic slowdown. Eating fast food is easy, but it's associated with inflammation and weight gain. Making success easier than failure isn't insulting to one's ego; it's not a sign of weakness, and it's not less impressive than "the hard way." It's just smarter.

How to Think About Weight Loss

These are a series of general mindsets for weight loss. Some are counterintuitive, and others are obvious. I'll explain why each is effective. If you get these wrong, you lose. If you get these right, you win.

Your Primary Goal Is Not Weight Loss: It's Behavior Change

When you want to lose weight, you shouldn't focus on how you look or what the scale says. These things matter for measuring objective progress, of course, but they are not your measure of *success*, because they are not the primary thing you're trying to change. This is akin to using a lever to move a heavy object. You can try to push the object directly, or you can use the lever's power of leverage to make the move far easier.

Behavior change is the lever of weight loss. Therefore, the measure of success with weight loss is the same as any other attempt to change your behavior: **To succeed with weight loss, you must change into the type of person who weighs less. If you do that, results will follow.**

This means that if during your journey you haven't lost weight but you've seen signs of behavioral change—whether it's a growing preference for eating salad, less resistance to exercising, or an increasing sense of self control—you're on your way to visible results. Behavior change always trumps weight change.

Do you think people would struggle if they could permanently, instantly, and visibly lose one pound of fat per hour spent on the treadmill? Of course not. To see that immediate cause and effect would be more than enough to motivate most people to lose all the weight they'd like to lose on a few marathon sessions.

Those who think they need results in order to motivate themselves to action have it exactly backwards. This viewpoint is why crash diets exist. Seeing 10 pounds lost in a week is supposed to trigger additional motivation to continue. This isn't an inherently terrible idea, as results are indeed motivating and motivation is a good thing. It is, however, completely unsustainable weight loss, and you're going to regain some or all of it back and take a motivation hit when you do, putting you in a worse position than when you started. The true formula to success is to take consistent action. Consistency creates habits, brings you results, and motivates you to continue. Results happen at the end of a process, not the beginning of it. As long as you maintain the process, you get the results. That's why we're going to master the process, which will *continuously* drive our results.

You're in Charge

Previous attempts to lose weight probably positioned you as a lowly pawn on the battlefield. The diet guru has sent in your instructions, and if you want to lose weight, you will follow the diet. Regardless of the diet's merit, this strips you of your sense of autonomy, and it makes it likely that you'll rebel.

With mini habits, you'll be designing your own battle plan. I'm giving you the information, materials, and ideas you need to succeed, but the style and exact plan of execution are completely up to you. You'll have options of different strategies, all of which will put you in a position of power, where you can leverage your easy choices into habits over time (the key to victory) and immediate results now (the key to morale). I'll tell you my favorite strategies and recommendations, but you know yourself and your life situation better than I do, so you will be making the final calls.

People can benefit from guidance, but they don't need to be controlled. No person loses weight and keeps it off by giving up control over their choices. Eventually, they will make their own decisions. With mini habits, you're in control from the start, so there's no transition to make. You will not lose your sense of self-rule.

I'll put it real-world terms: You will decide which days you overachieve with diet and exercise and which days you take a break and do the easy minimum. None of this takes away from your progress, because you'll make that every day, even on bad days. This is completely adaptable to your life and your whims, which is why mini habits are the king of consistency and the most powerful change strategy in the world.

Don't Be in A Rush
A study found that the best predictor of dropping out of weight loss treatment was high expectations for a lower BMI.[124] The more weight they expected to lose, the more likely they were to lose their goal instead.

Every person's mind and body are unique, and so the speed of weight loss is going to differ. Most weight loss books try to sell you on the speed of their method, taking advantage of people's desperation to "finally lose the weight." If a method doesn't consider permanent behavior change, it will *always* put you back to where you started, minus the cost of the book and the opportunity to have made real change in that time.

CRITICAL: The End Goal Is Not the Strategy
This is one of the most important concepts to learn, not only for weight loss, but for any goal you wish to pursue. Many people, when they set a goal, make their strategy the same as their end goal. For example, a person who wants to stop drinking soda may make their strategy "stop drinking soda." They assume it's best because it's the most obvious and visible strategy, but there are other strategies!

Every strategy you choose should be thoughtfully formed. If the best strategy for you happens to be the same as your end goal, then so be it. In my experience, the best strategy is rarely the most obvious one, because there are some counterintuitive aspects to behavior change. The futility of direct resistance is a great example of the obvious path being the inferior one.

To show you what I mean, here are eight (!) strategies you could use individually or in combination to stop drinking soda. The type of strategy is in parenthesis.

1. Stop drinking soda (direct resistance)
2. Limit soda consumption and pare down until eliminated ("weaning off")
3. Stop buying soda (starve the source/change the environment. There are sub-strategies for how to go about this as well.)
4. Create a consequence for drinking soda (negative

reinforcement)

5.   Choose a comparably enjoyable replacement drink and make it readily available (substitution)

6.   Delay drinking soda 10 minutes (establish control, reduce temptation, and wait out craving)

7.   Create an alternate path and pair it with a reward (neural pathway detour combined with positive reinforcement)

8.   Require yourself to drink a full glass of water before every soda (healthy obstacle and semi-substitute)

Isn't that refreshing? There are *at least* eight approaches to stop drinking soda. You're *not* trapped into trying and failing with the same one every time. In theory, any of them could work. In practice, some of them will work better, and some will depend on the person.

Since your strategy—not your desire—ultimately determines your success or failure, it's worth spending time to think about it. I've done that with the strategies I'll be recommending in this book, but don't think that my ideas are definitely the perfect strategy for you.

Addition over Subtraction
One of the most difficult things about weight loss is the common feeling that you have to give everything up. You feel like you have to watch less TV. You feel like you have to cut out all of your favorite junk foods. It seems boring, dull, and difficult.

What if instead of trying to cut back on all of the snack foods you eat, you simply required yourself to eat *more* healthy food? The more healthy food you eat, the more comfortable you'll be eating it. The problem isn't so much that people eat unhealthy food; it's that they *are trained to do it*. I eat unhealthy food on occasion, but my appetite for it is limited because I've practiced eating healthy food so much and now prefer it. I used to eat fast food almost every day, which only made me want to eat more of it. Every choice you make sets a precedent for the next time you're in that situation.

Dieting is deprivation, so it's a good thing we're not dieting. Successful weight loss is more about adding new and better things to your life than taking things away.

Don't Fear Food

When people diet, they "fear" certain foods that aren't part of their diet, whether it's bread or processed food or meat. They fear that they'll be tempted and eat it. When you fear something, you're admitting that it's more powerful than you in some way. We don't fear butterflies, because we know they can't and won't harm us.

Using fear as motivation seems powerful, but it puts you in a position of weakness. It also creates an all-or-nothing mindset. So, if you fear doughnuts (but really like them), you'll avoid them for as long as possible until your willpower breaks and you go back to your doughnut-eating ways. The more you go through this process, the more you'll reinforce the fear that you can't resist tempting foods.

Fear's all-or-nothing stakes damage your self-efficacy when things go poorly. Don't fear eating doughnuts. Strategically and calmly devise ways to eat fewer of them (we'll cover these in the Situational Strategies chapter). It's much easier to quit something with strategy than with emotion.

Lean toward Delaying Pleasure

Tomorrow does not exist. Today is all we'll ever have. We all know this, and it's good to be reminded of it. But there's an actionable takeaway here that's easy to miss, and that's to reverse your inclination. Instead of "I'll have soda now and drink water tomorrow," think "I'll drink water now and have a soda tomorrow." This is completely fine, even if you do drink a soda the next day.

It's satisfying to invest in yourself, knowing you have a reward waiting for you later. The anticipation of a reward is sometimes better than the actual reward itself. By delaying pleasure, you increase the length and intensity of your anticipatory rewards. and you'll end up doing the healthy thing more than planned. It works just as well for healthy food as it does for unhealthy food. Humans are good at procrastinating, and this is how to do it in a healthy way.

Delayed gratification is saying, "I know I can have this now, but I'm going to look forward to enjoying it later." Overeating food (typically of the ultra-processed variety) front-loads all the rewards you can stomach now (literally). This is actually an inferior strategy for maximizing your pleasure, because of the law of marginal utility.

I first learned about the law of marginal utility in Economics class, and my professor explained it well with a simple example: "You'll enjoy your first slice of pizza more than your second, and your second more than your fifth." You've probably noticed this phenomenon, not only in your eating, but in all of life. If you truly want to maximize your food rewards, you'd be better off not pushing the limits of your fullness. When you eat food beyond fullness, the only reward you gain is the taste of the food. It can be unenjoyable or even painful to digest food when you're already full. I could go into details like gas and bloating, but let's just skip that part.

I'm asking you to eat smarter and enjoy your food in a different way, not suffer for weight loss. The same suggestion (don't overeat) is often framed in such a way that makes you feel deprived for doing it, as if it's a sacrifice you must make to lose weight.

Humans need rewards, and we will get them however we can. For lasting success, we must aim to live a rewarding lifestyle that results in weight loss. As you get better at delaying gratification, you will make more of the right decisions now and feel rewarded *from that*. Afterwards, additional gratification will come in the form of the pleasures you delayed and a healthier and more attractive body.

Don't make this a hard rule: just attempt to lean toward delaying pleasure and doing the healthier thing today. There's a fine line between direct resistance and leaning toward delayed gratification, but it's absolutely critical to be on the right side of it. You'll know which side of it you're on, based on the amount of resistance you feel. If you feel a lot of resistance, it's because you're resisting too hard. Relax. Lower the stakes.

Present-Day Thinking

One of the most difficult aspects of weight loss is the weight of the past. If you've been overweight for a while, you may feel ashamed about your lifestyle or your weight. I invite you to drop that burden. You don't deserve it or need it. It doesn't benefit you, and it's actually illogical to let it influence you.

Consider that this moment forward is unwritten, and therefore it is *objectively* neutral. You can live any number of different ways from here, which is why dwelling on the past isn't merely a waste of time, but also a hindrance to forward progress.

Mutual funds will often give the disclaimer that "past results do not guarantee future performance." The same is true for our lives, whether we've had excellent or poor results in the past. For those who have a past full of regrets and poor choices, this is freedom. For those who have been doing well, it's a reminder to keep going. You can't change the past, so don't worry about it.

You're Training

One of the biggest mistakes that nearly every person makes when trying to lose weight is in the perspective of what they're doing. If you're going to try mini habits for weight loss, you'll do things differently, and you're going to love the change! Why?

You're not being punished. You're not "making sacrifices" to lose weight.

Those are losing perspectives. What do top athletes do? Train. What do top writers do? Write. What does anyone successful do to get where they are? Practice their craft until they succeed.

Just like some people are born with athletic genes and some people learn to golf at an early age, some of us are genetically given slenderness (regardless of lifestyle) or have learned to manage our weight. Many others have been put in the "Western Lifestyle Program," a weight-gaining system that works extremely well. You are going to retrain your brain and body to be healthier and lighter.

If you don't like your current weight, but you like your current lifestyle, you've got a choice to make, because your lifestyle IS your weight. Lifestyle and weight are white on rice and cold on ice. They're permanently bonded and inseparable. Lifestyle isn't all-or-nothing, though. Just because you've changed to generally eat well and stay active doesn't mean you can't also eat chocolate truffles, drink socially, or binge-watch a TV series. Anyone who tells you these things are "forbidden for weight loss" is wrong on multiple levels.

The healthy lifestyle is extremely enjoyable, and I'm not talking about the health or weight benefits. To show you what I mean, here is an example of a positive chain of a healthy lifestyle: better nutrition leads to better sleep, which leads to fewer cravings, which leads to better eating habits, all of which lead to more energy, which leads to a more active lifestyle, which leads to improved physical and mental performance, which leads to more confidence and success, which leads to more money, which leads to a Ferrari. Better nutrition leads to a Ferrari? That's unlikely. Even so, the chain effect of healthy living is powerful in surprising ways. You may not get a Ferrari from eating blueberries, but you will notice some unexpected tangential changes when living healthier.

Athletes have some of the strictest diets and training programs, and many of them enjoy every minute of it. People get addicted to going to the gym. People lust for salads. This is not impossible for anyone, it's just foreign to most.

Choose Boundaries over Rules, Identity over Slavery, and "Don't" over "Can't"

What's the first thing a person thinks when they try to lose weight?

I can't eat junk food. I have to eat more vegetables.

It sounds correct and innocent enough, but this is an awful way of thinking about weight loss. First, notice the loss of control in the language. I *can't*, I *have to*. These are phrases we use when we have no choice; these are phrases we used when our parents told us we couldn't spend the night at a friend's house.

"Sorry, James, Mom says I can't sleep over tonight."
~ An actual quote from a young, sad Stephen (I still love you, Mom).

In contrast, what does a non-smoking adult say when offered a cigarette?

"No thanks, I don't smoke."

The child is not in control of his situation. The adult is.

Consider that "can't" is more an appeal to authority than a personal decision to change. Like in the child's case, he wants to sleep over, but he can't, because his parents said so. When an adult tries this "can't strategy" with dieting and they realize that they are in fact still the decision-maker, it's really easy to break that rule.

There's science, too. Vanessa Patrick and Henrik Hagtvedt gathered 120 students and asked them to quantify their desire for healthy eating (on a 1-9 scale).[125] Some students were told to use "I don't eat X" and others "I can't eat X" to combat temptation to eat unhealthy snacks.

After this, participants were moved to what they thought was an unrelated study, and, once they handed in their questionnaire from that, they were offered a chocolate bar or "healthy" granola bar. A piece of fruit would be a better fit as a healthy snack, but regardless, the study results *were* quite interesting.

They saw 64% of the "I don't" group choose granola bars and the rest choose chocolate bars. Only 39% of the "I can't" group chose granola bars.

The reason "don't" works so much better than "can't" is because it's identity-based, rather than a superficial attempt to control your behavior. In the study conductors' words: "Since the 'don't' frame suggests a stable and unchanging stance that invokes the self ('this is who I am'), it is more effective when goal focus is internal and related to the self (I don't eat fast food)."[126]

The takeaway: identity-based decisions EMPOWER your internal long-term goals (such as those in weight loss); following baseless rules of a "can't" nature WEAKEN you and activate your rebellious side.

If you decide not to have cake and someone pushes you to have some or asks you why you won't, please don't say that you're on a diet. Don't say that you "can't have any." That makes you look and feel deprived. Instead, say that you don't want any. That makes you look and feel powerful. See the difference?

As surprising as it sounds, it's perfectly okay to turn down unhealthy food because you don't want it, rather than because you're "watching your weight." Society places a lot of pressure on us to succumb to processed foods, but they're not as appealing when you consider the ingredients and the effect they have on your body. You may not yet see processed food in this way, but when you train yourself to enjoy real food with mini habits, you're going to feel and look better, and your preferences will change. The person who eats low-quality food isn't aware of how great they'd feel eating healthy food.

This is not to say that you won't ever eat French fries again. I'm the weird guy who offers his friends carrots for snacking and fresh fruit for dessert when they come over. I still consume things like French fries, hamburgers, wine, beer, and pizza. Rarely, I'll even drink soda, even though I hate what it's done to human health. Nothing except artificial sweeteners and trans fats are completely off limits for me. I don't have rules saying what I can and can't eat. I don't eat unhealthy foods very often because I've changed my identity. You can do it too.

Don't Assign Morality to Your Food Choices

Once you make food a moral battle, you weaken. Eating certain types of food doesn't make you good or bad. It doesn't make you inferior or superior to anyone else. We eat food to survive. Some food is more nutritious than other food, but it all (mostly) works to keep us alive. Did you know there's a woman who has eaten nothing but pizza for many years?

I eat a very healthy diet relative to most people, but it makes me no better or worse than anyone else. It makes me no better than I was when I ate fast food all the time in college. I have more energy now, and my diet has improved my health, but our value as people has *nothing* to do with what we eat.

You know how people will say, "Oh, I'm so bad," before eating an entire chocolate cake? That's making food into a moral battle. It is saying that you're doing something wrong. Can you guess what emotions that generates? Guilt and shame. Whoops.

Food choices aren't good and bad. They are beneficial or harmful to your health, well-being, and weight loss goal. When you eat a doughnut, you needn't feel as if you betrayed your best friend. You needn't feel like you're a bad person. Instead, be aware that you chose to eat food for entertainment over sustenance. Be aware that you likely added a bit of fat to your belly. There's nothing *wrong* with it, but there *are* consequences.

Forget the Congruency Mindset and Binge on Healthy Food

Have you ever thought about why you're more likely to binge-eat potato chips than broccoli? You might think it's because chips are tastier and easier to consume in bulk, and that may be true to some extent, but there's another, more dangerous reason.

People are less likely to eat significant amounts of healthy food because of their mindset. Chips are known to be a weight-gaining food, as they're high carb, high fat, high calorie, and not very satiating. So when a person begins eating chips, they see it as a "poor choice." Since we tend to desire congruency, and overeating chips is a combination of two weight loss mistakes (eating a weight-gaining food and eating too much of it), it's mentally satisfying, albeit disappointing later, to act in congruence with the "bad label." We've all probably thought, "Well, I've made this mistake, so I might as well finish making it."

When we eat broccoli, we're cognizant that we're doing a good thing for our body, and eating an excessive amount of food would seem to "go against" our good decision. Since we're being "good" at the time, we don't want to overeat and tarnish our good deed. But it's almost impossible to overeat healthy food and unwise to moderate it artificially. If you artificially limit the amount of broccoli you can eat now, you're going to eat more of something else later. This isn't to say that you MUST eat a lot of broccoli. It's to show you why you don't need to fear overeating healthy food.

One reason real food triggers satiety before ultra-processed food is because of a concept called sensory specific satiety. Sensory specific satiety is the term for losing the desire for a particular food after consuming a certain amount of it. For me, egg nog and chocolate fudge trigger my sensory specific satiety very quickly. They taste delicious, but they're so strong and "in your face" that I can't handle too much.

Food scientists know about this phenomenon, and they've found a way around it. If a food or drink is nuanced with different flavors, we can consume (much) more of it. Did you know that soft drink flavors are *engineered* to be pleasant, but nuanced and not too strong to avoid triggering your sensory specific satiety so that you'll drink more? It's true.

When you are near healthy food, eat as much of it as you want. It will feel strange to mix large portion sizes with healthy food choices because common wisdom says to eat less, but overeating is *rarely* an issue with fruits and vegetables. The 24-year study with over 100,000 participants I mentioned earlier found that the most weight loss was associated *per serving* of fruit, meaning that additional servings of fruit meant more weight loss.[127]

I regularly binge on frozen fruit (typically mangoes and blueberries) covered with cinnamon for dessert, and it usually amounts to only about 200 to 300 calories before I'm completely satisfied.

Don't Aim to Lose Weight, Aim to Not Gain it
A study on obese Black women found that the women had better weight

loss results when they aimed for weight maintenance rather than weight loss.[128] Attempting to "lose weight" makes you think you have to do more than you actually do. It suggests that you are "behind" and need to do something extra, which isn't true. It leads to the scarcity mindset and suggests that you eat less food (both of which are weight-gaining perspectives). Trying not to gain weight correctly puts your focus on things like the type of food you're eating and not stuffing yourself (rather than aiming for a deficit).

Heavy Thoughts to Avoid

There are certain thoughts that practically add pounds all by themselves, because of how much they affect your behavior. Don't think these thoughts if you want to lose weight.

1. *I can trust this food.* People place too much trust in the food system. It's important to remember that people who sell you food are running a business, and your health is *not even close* to the top of their concerns list. This includes "diet" products, as the perfect "diet product" is one that you think works, but doesn't.

When something is labeled "diet," it often means it contains artificial sweeteners. On examining data from a 9-year study in San Antonio, researchers found that those who consumed 21 artificially sweetened beverages (ASBs) per week were almost twice as likely to be overweight or obese. Those who consumed artificial sweetened beverages experienced a 47% greater weight gain than those who did not. "Significant positive dose-response relationship emerged between baseline ASB consumption and all outcome measures."[129] Another study found that artificially sweetened beverages may even promote weight gain more than sugar sweetened beverages.[130]

2. *I deserve a treat.* Dogs get treats. Humans get rewards. We need a broader term than treat, because we can reward ourselves in many different ways besides eating. Finding alternative rewards is an essential part of transforming habits like overeating and stress eating.

3. *This meal is a small exception.* Special occasions and exceptions are the enemy of consistency, and that means they're the enemy of successful weight loss. Remember the power of small compounded changes that we

discussed? This applies to small *exceptions*, too. The innocent-sounding "just this once" has ruined lives by creating or sustaining addictions. It's necessary to understand the compounding power of small directional shifts in your life for better AND for worse. Never discount the helpfulness of eating a carrot, or the possible damage from saying "just this once." (Note: Mini habits minimize the need or desire for exceptions.)

4. *If other people are doing it, it's acceptable.* Social eating dynamics are a big reason why people struggle with their weight. It's a triple whammy:

- We want to fit in.
- We don't want to offend anyone.
- We assume that other people take care of themselves to a reasonable degree.

Imagine you're eating dinner, and everyone orders a cheesecake to share. In this situation, you don't really want the cheesecake because you know it contains artificial ingredients, is highly processed, and the taste isn't worth it to you at this time. If it were just you, you'd turn it down easily. But everyone encourages you to try a bite, they're all enjoying it, and it seems that they're reasonably healthy and having fun, so what's the harm?

The harm isn't the individual case of eating a little bit of cheesecake. It's that you are allowing your decisions to be controlled by something outside of you. If you eat cheesecake or anything else, be sure that you're the one making the decision and don't be afraid to say no.

It's more important to uphold your values than to be courteous 100% of the time; it's okay to be rude if you're protecting your values. Some people will disagree with that, because they believe that social etiquette rules all. If someone is so offended that you won't eat cheesecake or drink alcohol with them, you are the one who should be offended that they don't respect your desires and values. True friends will support your quest to become a better person, and not get upset if you refuse to consume unhealthy food with them. It's critical to be able to say no, because, if you can't, you'll be at the mercy of other people's ideas for life.

In the United States, it's "normal" for people to drink soda with every meal. To be at a healthy weight in a country with a population that is

110

70% overweight, you have to be different from most people. We're influenced by those we spend time with, and within that truth is a good piece of advice: If you can find them, seek out and spend time with people who live a healthy lifestyle.

Even with the strategies I'm going to give to you, it will remain extremely difficult to change if your environment is filled with people with unhealthy habits who always eat unhealthy food. Environment is one of the most powerful forces in our lives. If you find yourself struggling, take a close look at how your environment is driving your behavior.

5. *Dancing for 30 seconds right now won't help me lose weight.* If you want to gain weight, make your standard for exercise and healthy eating so high that you can only meet it when you've prepared extensively for it. When you put healthy living on a pedestal, you'll do it less.

Yes, exercise is important. Yes, it can help you lose weight in the long term. But no, you don't need to do it impressively in clean 30-minute segments. Make exercise a common thing, dance around for a few seconds in the same way you'd grab a snack. Do a push-up (or a few) while waiting for the microwave to finish. A low bar to entry increases the number of entries. Right now, stand up and move around for 10 seconds. It's just 10 seconds. You don't have to do Tai Chi if you're in the airport. You can simply get up and stretch or walk around for 10 seconds. If you can do this, you can succeed with mini habits. Read on when you finish.

If you haven't done it yet and are feeling resistance to doing it, explore what you're feeling. Your objections are probably about it not being good enough, that it's inconvenient with no payoff, that you'd do it if you were in a different situation, and probably a vague feeling that you'd be better off not doing it. This is because you haven't practiced doing such small behaviors and seen the payoff. When something is foreign to you, your subconscious will throw up these "smokescreen" excuses. Just this once, force yourself to do it as an experiment. It's just 10 seconds. After you finish, compare the experience to your thoughts prior to doing it. At worst, you'll see it as a neutral experience.

Did you feel your heart rate or alertness slightly increase? This is good. This little bit of movement is good enough, because it's better than sitting for 10 seconds. It doesn't prevent you from doing more, but it does make you far more likely to do more now or in the future. Every time you demonstrate your ability to take a small positive step like this, you decrease your resistance to further steps now or later.

6. *In order to lose weight, I've got to do something big. I've got to make a huge change.* Similar to the previous point, those who put the most pressure on themselves to make the biggest changes are the ones who fail most frequently. In a previously mentioned study, the best predictor of dropping out of weight loss treatment was high expectations for a lower BMI.[131] The more weight they expected to lose, the less weight they lost.

The people who succeed financially are rarely those who receive windfall gains; they're the people who methodically save and invest their money, growing their net worth steadily. In the same way, those who successfully lose weight don't do it in 10 days; they gradually change their behavior over time and their body steadily improves. As with the wealthy, no individual day's progress is electrifying, but the overall result will be.

7. *I need to eat less.* Careful with this one! This is one of the counterintuitive aspects of weight loss. It seems smart to think this way, but it activates your scarcity instincts. Scarce things are irresistible to us. When your life revolves around the amount of food you're eating, you're a slave to it, not a master of it. In the long term, it means you'll probably overeat.

To lose weight, you need to have a mindset of abundance. Think: *I have enough food to eat. This amount of food is satisfying. I've had plenty, and my next meal is coming soon.* This will encourage you to stop at satiety rather than careen into belt-snapping territory because you've made food seem scarce and rare.

Shame Is the Obstacle, Not the Solution

Shame is different from guilt. Shame is inward, and guilt is outward. As Joseph Burgo, PhD, puts it, "Guilt and shame sometimes go hand in hand; the same action may give rise to feelings of both shame and guilt, where the former reflects how we feel about ourselves and the latter involves an awareness that our actions have injured someone else. In other words, shame relates to self, guilt to others."[132] Shame is the feeling that you've let yourself down, that you've been "bad."

When you feel ashamed about doing something, you are much more likely to do that same thing again. Shame cycles are devastating and persistent, because shame weakens the self. When you're weak, you're vulnerable to making decisions you'll feel shameful about later. It's the opposite of the prototypical commander, captain, king, or queen, who makes firm, confident decisions from their position of strength.

When I'm feeling shameful about playing video games and let it fester, to put it eloquently, it makes me feel like a pile of poop. Then I'll want to do something fun to make me feel better and distract me from my feelings, something like playing video games. So, by feeling shame about playing video games too much, I'm more likely to play them more. Ouch.

Shame Is Pain

Shame is a form of emotional pain, and, like all pain, its purpose is to deter the behavior that causes it. Shame rarely works as intended, because it weakens us. The weaker you are, the more pain you'll feel, and, when it's too much to handle, it leads to the same comforting and distracting behaviors that caused your initial shame, and the cycle begins. Therefore, shame doesn't work very well to deter *shameful behaviors*.

Shame weakens us, making us become more pliable to our environment, so a person *can* become a more willing puppet to another party (or dieting system) through shame, but, aside from harming the individual in ways more important than weight, this offers no chance at sustaining weight loss, which must come from an individual's inner strength and choices. When shame is self-inflicted, like when you feel it before, during, or after eating something, it only harms you, your confidence, and your sense of self-worth and self-respect, all of which are far more devastating to your goal of weight loss than the most fattening food. **Shame motivates us to avoid behaviors that cause further shame, which is useful in theory, but it is an even more powerful destroyer of self-respect, which is why it seems right and works wrong.**

We need to reduce feelings of shame as much as possible, and the upcoming strategies are designed with that in mind.

Autonomy

What's the difference between a person who exercises because they enjoy it and a person who does it because it's a part of their "15 Pounds in 15 Days" bootcamp? Autonomy.

Autonomy in psychology is defined as making choices according to your own free will. It's a critical but chronically overlooked factor in self-improvement and goal-setting. Autonomy is important for one simple reason—we all want to (and do) run our own show. Sometimes we give up our sense of autonomy for the promise of a specific result. There's one serious problem with that. **You can only lose your sense of autonomy, not your actual autonomy.**

What happens when you're told that you must exercise until exhaustion and eat less food to lose weight? You lose your sense of autonomy, but not your actual autonomy. In time, you will rest and eat as before.

While you can suppress your sense of autonomy to "follow the system" for a while, you're eventually going to take control again. This is the calculation we get wrong, isn't it? We commit to a difficult workout or diet program and think we can just "suck it up" until we get the result we want, but at some point, we will officially take back the control that we pretended to give up.

This isn't limited to ideas we read from others, either. You can lose your sense of autonomy from a goal that *you* set previously. For example, let's say that Jane decides for her New Year's Resolution that she will lose 100 pounds by exercising two hours per day. Ten days later, Jane wants to rest because her knee hurts and she's so sore she can barely move, but she *feels controlled* by the public decree she made on top of the dining room table after her ~~second~~ sixth glass of champagne. Jane's going to quit her plan altogether. And what will she feel at that point? Relief. Freedom. After such a letdown and failure, why does Jane feel relieved? Because she's regained her sense of autonomy.

People receive undeserved criticism when they stop dieting. Others say, "You should have stuck with the program." They imply that it's better to be thin and miserable than overweight and free. But we'll never stick to a dieting program, because our freedom means more to us than anything else.

The Two Levels of Autonomy

The best goal strategies will not only protect your sense of autonomy, but also enhance it. This is tricky because autonomy exists at two levels, conscious and subconscious. The opposite of autonomy is slavery, and here's what it looks like at the two levels.

Conscious Slavery Example: You want to lose weight and decide to avoid eating cake, but you see a slice of cake and eat it. Your conscious desire (lose weight, avoid cake) was controlled by your subconscious desire (eat cake). You'll feel like a slave to the cake.

Subconscious Slavery Example: You want to lose weight and decide to avoid eating cake, and when you see a slice of cake, you resist it. Now your subconscious desire (eat cake) is being controlled by your conscious desire (lose weight, avoid cake). You'll feel deprived because you want the cake.

It seems like a lose-lose situation, doesn't it? Whether you eat the cake or not, some part of you is going to feel controlled. Anyone who has attempted to lose weight is familiar with this predicament, because dieting provides people with a temporary way to make the healthy choices to get the results they want. Until their motivation and willpower are exhausted, they can live in such a way to lose weight (their conscious desire). But our subconscious is powerful, and it will not allow itself to be controlled for long. Your cravings will get stronger. Your ability to resist will weaken. The conscious mind wins in the short term, but the subconscious wins in the long term.

The only lasting, permanent solution for this conundrum is to align your conscious and subconscious to desire the same thing. What if you wanted to avoid cake to lose weight consciously AND didn't have a strong urge to eat it subconsciously? That's now a win-win situation, because neither part of you desires the cake. This puts us into habit formation territory, which is the practice of shaping the subconscious to mirror your conscious preferences.

To successfully form a habit or change an old one, you must be consistent with the change for an extended amount of time. A 16-year cake-eating habit will not go away after 10 days of starving yourself on green smoothies. You won't likely go from a couch potato to a lifelong fitness freak in 30 days either. Both of those strategies, as popular as they are, strangle your subconscious's sense of freedom. We choose these plans because they align with our conscious interests. But ignore your subconscious desires at the peril of your goals, because if you fight it, you will lose. You may win for 10 or 30 days, but we've covered the folly of temporary weight loss. To win, you need to change your subconscious preferences, not declare war on them.

The *Mini Habits for Weight Loss* strategy is designed to preserve and protect your sense of conscious and subconscious freedom. When you're in charge, and when your strategy is flexible enough to adapt to your life and subconscious desires, the gradual changes you make can last a lifetime.

The best strategies for big changes are adaptable to you. The worst strategies for big changes tell you to suck it up and follow directions if you want results. If you're mailing a letter, sure, follow directions, but if you're attempting to overhaul the way you've lived for decades, you're going to need more than a list of foods, an exercise plan, and a pat on the back. You need a strategy that can meet you where you are subconsciously and integrate changes into your life as seamlessly as possible.

Now it's time to delve into that strategy. We'll begin with food.

6
Food Strategy

**Here's a List of Foods to Eat and Avoid.
Just Kidding. Let's Do Something Smarter.**

*"Between stimulus and response there is a space. In that space
is our power to choose our response. In our response lies our
growth and our freedom."*
~ Viktor Frankl

Do Not Ban Junk Food

If you want to give this strategy a try, you are allowed to eat any food whenever you want. No limits. Nothing is forbidden. You can eat unhealthy food. There's no calorie counting. It's all up to your discretion.

We're using a pro-healthy-food strategy, rather than the common anti-unhealthy-food strategy. When you rely on food avoidance rules, your willpower and motivation to adhere to them will almost certainly fail you at some point, and then it gets awkward. Once you've failed, do you reinstate the rule immediately? Do you try a different plan? Many people give up once they "break the seal" and eat even more forbidden food than usual.

Food bans actually make the banned food more desirable in the long term, as we're psychologically drawn to things we can't have. A formal ban also suggests that this food is so desirable that your only chance is to force yourself to stay away from it. It's the wrong approach, because it increases the perceived value of low-quality food.

The true goal is to eat healthy food, anyway. Eating is mostly a zero sum game, in that if you're eating healthy food all day, you won't have room left to fit in other food. Some people fear eating healthy food, thinking they'll continue to eat the same amount of unhealthy food and therefore eat even more calories. This is not true to a relevant extent, because healthy food WILL take up some room in your stomach and it's very satiating on a per calorie basis.

Besides, cutting out unhealthy food 100% with no exceptions is not sustainable or desirable for most people. It may sound crazy, but it's better to fully allow junk food so that you'll be able to eat *less* of it long term.

You probably have some questions about this approach, such as: *How is this different from the typical person not on a diet who already allows unhealthy food and eats it excessively?*

Live Between Banning and Mindless Eating

To control food intake, people initially try banning it, causing them to cycle between total abstinence and out-of-control bingeing. You will gain control of your diet by finding a sustainable place between those extremes. **Whatever you attempt to do in order to improve your body must be completely and unquestionably sustainable.** Trying to do too much will make it worse.

The *New York Times* said of Danny Cahill, former contestant of *The Biggest Loser*: "Mr. Cahill, 46, said his weight problem began when he was in the third grade. He got fat, then fatter. He would starve himself, and then eat a whole can of cake frosting with a spoon. Afterward, he would cower in the pantry off the kitchen, feeling overwhelmed with shame."[133] This type of shame- and deprivation-driven cycle is not only a horrible experience, but it's also an extremely poor strategy that results in binges and a waistline that expands like a scared pufferfish. For food and life in general, the harder you directly try to suppress your desires, the stronger they'll become.

A no-cake run that ends in a cake binge is far more weight-gaining than not dieting at all. On the other hand, consistently choosing to eat cake less often or in smaller portions can result in a big, permanent, and positive change that can be further improved. Also, when you *consciously and mindfully* eat cake, you might decide in hindsight that it isn't worth it, and that could help you choose differently next time. The transition from a person who always eats unhealthy food to a person who allows it but usually chooses not to have it is first mindfulness and then new habits.

A great "side effect" of having mini habits is increased mindfulness of your food and movement choices every day. Being mindful of your behavior means you'll be better able to control it. You'll know your triggers. You'll be cognizant of what you need to do.

Even if you do just one minute of jogging in place per day, you'll be more mindful of exercise. Even if you only drink one glass of water at a specified time every day, you'll be more mindful of your subsequent beverage choices. One mini habit in your breakfast routine will make you more mindful about your other meals. If there was only one change a person could choose to make for their weight loss journey, the right choice would be increased mindfulness. It helps change bad, mindless habits back into decisions we make and keeps us looking for other opportunities to make progress.

When you combine mindfulness about your food decisions with a positive drive forward to eat real foods, the effect is a small and consistent change in the right direction. The power in this change is exceptionally more potent than it will ever seem, because, unlike temporary change, sustainable changes compound over time.

No Limits Means Smarter Choices

I allow myself to eat unhealthy food in any amount, but rarely *choose* to do so. Because of gradual changes I've made to my diet, I now generally prefer the benefits and taste of unprocessed, nature-made food.

One day, I ate at a Greek restaurant, and my side choice was fries or a salad. This is a classic weight loss decision between foods at two ends of the spectrum. (I don't need to lose weight, but my desire to be healthy rivals the desire of people wanting to lose weight, so it was a similar situation.) I had been eating very healthy food for a while, so I decided to splurge and order the fries. But then I started fantasizing about the salad. This isn't a joke, it's a true story. I ended up getting the salad when I planned to get the fries, and this sort of thing now happens frequently in my life (and need I remind you, I am a former candy and fast food addict).

This is exactly the reverse of what typically happens with people who have unhealthy eating habits, isn't it? They *try* to order the salad, but fantasize about the fries and get those instead. It's no different from my salad story; it's just the opposite habit driving the decision.

If I had told myself that I absolutely can't have fries because they're unhealthy, the little bit of desire I had for them would have increased dramatically. It would have been a choice between the boring salad I'm "supposed to eat" and the forbidden, delicious fries that I can't have. See how that perspective pushes us in the wrong direction?

Don't underestimate the power of habit to change your preferences. Notice that my salad story above is not about me overcoming an insatiable desire for fries and heroically choosing the salad. I'm not lying to you when I say I'm lazier and have lower willpower than most people. I didn't overcome *anything* and I'm not a hero, I just preferred the salad, which exemplifies why successful weight loss is not a willpower fight.

It is possible for you to plan on eating junk food and desire healthier food when the time comes. If people could fully understand and experience how much easier and more effective it is to target their habits to change their preferences than to fight themselves, they'd drop the diets and cleanses and prioritize habit formation. I hope this book helps make that happen.

Habits are our preferences, and, if we're smart, we can shape them to work for us instead of against us. Contrast the effortlessness of habit-driven behavior to the person who tries to win through sheer willpower, suppressing their food choices and calorie consumption for days, weeks, or months. Those who attempt to win through brute force work much harder, but those who leverage habits work smarter to get much farther.

Take 100% Responsibility

Self-responsibility is dying because of all the systems we rely upon today. We eat the food produced by the food systems in place. When attempting weight loss, we eat things labeled "diet."

These systems take away our control, which can limit our sense of responsibility for our lives. There's nothing wrong with following a system *if the system brings you the right results.* If a system does not produce the right results, it's our job to get out of it and take back control and responsibility.

Ideally, we'd accept 100% responsibility at all times for all things, but it takes time and energy (two limited resources) to assume full responsibility for something, so we end up selectively choosing what we're going to focus on.

So many people are overweight today because they rely on the world's food systems, which are highly obesogenic. The diet and weight loss systems that are supposed to "fix" the problem are even more broken and ineffective. With two failing systems, we need to take 100% of our responsibility back to get healthy and lose weight.

The way to take back responsibility is to question everything. Is food coloring safe to eat? What does potassium sorbate do in the human body? What happens to oils when they're heated to high temperatures? Will this diet product actually help me or just give me a short-term result and false hope? Is this fruit smoothie really 100% raw fruit blended up, with nothing else added? These are questions that the typical person does not ask, does not care to ask, or doesn't have the time, energy, or expertise to answer. These questions matter, not just for being at a healthy weight, but for being in good health and minimizing your risk for disease.

Many see good health as the single most important part of a high-quality life. Those already in decent to good health might not say that, but those in poor health understand its supreme importance. That's just to say that this particular area is worth taking full responsibility over, regardless of where you currently stand in weight and health.

Think about this: Dieting trains people to give up their responsibility by following a set of rules. This book will arm you with strategies and ask you to take full responsibility for your food choices outside of your daily mini habits. Those who take back responsibility and stop pressuring themselves to eat perfectly and instead look to make small, sustainable, and reasonable changes will succeed.

Take full responsibility for your weight and health from this point on, and never give it away. If we could trust things labeled low-calorie, diet, low-fat, no carbs, etc., then we wouldn't have to think about food and we'd all be thin. The next section is called "How They Trick Ya." You'll see why those who trust food corporations end up sick and fat.

Some people see the word "diet" on a food product, assume it helps them lose weight, and drop their responsibility on the spot. They will continue to gain weight. There is no regulation for labeling a product "diet," and even if there were, it would probably be based on the calorie content of the product, not the total weight impact of the product.

The Modern Challenge of Healthy Living
The current difficulty of living a healthy lifestyle is the unfortunate result of what many societies worldwide are becoming and have become. American society in particular has demanded convenience and branding over simple healthy eating. We the people are to blame, just as much as the corporations. No-added-sugar products don't typically sell as well as those with added sugar, which is why those products are now hard to find. That's the sign of an entire society not taking responsibility for their food choices, because, if taste is the highest or only factor, high sugar products will sell the best (and they do).

While making it easier to live well is the basis of our strategy, taking full responsibility for yourself is the one thing you must do that cannot be made easier. Nobody else can do it for you. You must own what you eat and own how active you are. How can anyone not eat healthy food if they make it the *most important thing?* Many have delegated their personal responsibility for their health and well-being to grocery stores, restaurants, and the government—they are too busy making money and governing, respectively, to take responsibility for individual health.

If you take responsibility (which, in most cases, is as easy as being generally skeptical of food and looking at ingredients to know what you're eating), and set up some mini habits, you will succeed. But you need to know what you're up against. Food is big business, and therefore, deception is rampant. Let's talk about how they deceive us.

Know How They Trick Ya

If a food corporation uses phrasing that seems healthy but has a potential loophole, their product is almost certainly unhealthy and to be avoided. Sometimes, actually healthy qualities will be listed, but it doesn't mean it's a healthy product, as processed food can hit you from so many angles. In this section, I'll give you a few examples of trickery used to deceive customers into thinking a food is healthier than it really is.

If you read any of these on a package, pull the alarm, because a company is probably trying to trick you into making a poor decision. Every time you pick up a food item, skip the branding on front, flip it over, and look at the ingredients. Here's some reasons why you shouldn't trust everything you read on the front packaging. There are far more examples than the ones listed below, but these will give you an idea of what we're up against.

100% Wheat!
What a person might think: 100% wheat! Perfect! This is the type of healthy wheat product I should be eating.
What it means: The product does not contain millet or quinoa (useless information). Saying 100% wheat does NOT mean that the wheat is *whole*, that there aren't other ingredients, and that it hasn't been refined and processed into oblivion.

Multigrain!
What a person might think: Yes! A lot of healthy grains for me!

What it means: More than one grain is used. They can still be refined, devoid of nutritional content, and doctored with caramel coloring to make them look like whole grains. A very popular sandwich chain has a nine-grain bread with the first two ingredients being "whole wheat flour and "enriched flour." Enriched flour means refined white flour. Then, it goes on to list the other eight grains in the 2% or less category. It's basically a combination of whole wheat and white bread, with trace amounts of other grains. Technically, it contains nine grains, but aside from some whole wheat, it contains more white bread than the other eight grains combined! It's white bread wearing healthy-looking make-up.

Made with whole grains!
What a person might think: This product is 100% whole grains!
What it means: Whole grains are somewhere on the list of ingredients, probably right after the refined grains (which make up most of the food). The magical phrase to look for when it comes to bread or pasta is 100% whole grain. That's what you want to see. Anything else is a loophole. And of course, any ultra-processed foods, even those made with 100% whole grains, are still not ideal.

Made with (100%) real cheese!
What a person might think: This product is mostly real cheese.
Wheat it means: Real cheese is used, but it might account for 2% of the total product. This is common practice with cheese crackers, which contain a little bit of cheese and a lot of refined flour.

Low Fat!
What a person might think: This product is healthy and good for weight loss.
What it (probably) means: High sugar! High sodium! High in preservatives! Highly processed! Highly unhealthy! Highly profitable!

Extra Virgin Olive Oil!
Olive oil's health benefits are top tier when it comes to fats, and it's an ideal choice for weight loss. If you're after the health benefits, you should only consider buying extra virgin olive oil, which is made by crushing olives (other oils are often heated and processed with chemicals). Since extra virgin olive oil has become a big business in high demand, it has attracted corruption, and your bottle of extra virgin olive oil might not be so pure. Whereas the other prior cases were misleading, but technically true, this is a case of pure deception.

UC Davis collaborated with the International Oil Council to analyze 186 olive oil samples in two studies over two years. In the second study, they found that, of the five top-selling imported bottles of extra virgin olive oil in the United States, 73% of samples failed the IOC sensory panel. "Sensory defects are indicators that these samples are oxidized, of poor quality, and/or adulterated with cheaper refined oils."[134] As for the latter, extra virgin olive oil is sometimes mixed with cheaper, unhealthy, refined oils like canola or soybean oil. They also tested the fatty acid profile to distinguish real olive oil from other nut/seed oils.

If you just want to know the brands that passed the tests as real, pure, and quality 100% extra virgin olive oil, the two brands that passed all tests in all 18 samples were California Olive Ranch and Cobram Estate. Lucini was third, with 16 of 18 samples passing the tests. Consumer reports did a similar study, with very few brands making the mark (once again, California Olive Ranch and Lucini were among the winners).[135]

Based on these results, I decided to purchase a bottle of California Olive Ranch extra virgin olive oil. It smelled like no other olive oil I've tried—very rich and aromatic, and clearly the real deal. The last oil I tried was an organic Mediterranean blend and it didn't have that type of rich aroma. I highly recommend going with one of the above-listed brands for your olive oil. I have no affiliation with California Olive Ranch or any incentive to promote them or any other olive oil company. Honest companies deserve to be talked about.

Change Your Food Preferences

When a soccer player wants to improve his kicking mechanics, he doesn't slap himself in the face if he kicks the ball incorrectly; *he practices kicking it correctly*. If he can learn the correct kicking technique and continue to practice that, it will become a stronger habit than any of his former poor techniques, and he'll have improved his game. This is a simple, obvious, and straightforward process. But how many people when dieting try to use guilt and punishment to motivate themselves to eat the *right* things? How many people make their food choices into a moral battle between "good" and "bad" foods, rather than just practicing healthy eating?

Perhaps it's hard to see that eating is like every other behavior, in that it's tied to habitual processes. The way to change your diet is to practice the new diet you'd like to have, not to forbid certain foods and hope you can resist. That bears repeating. **You change your diet by practicing the new diet you'd like to have, not by forbidding unhealthy foods.**

Let's assume that you're currently a candy-eating, soda-guzzling, fast food hall-of-famer. Do you really think that avoiding these foods is the answer? All that would do is leave you hungry and frustrated. If instead you learn to enjoy healthy foods, you'll begin to prefer them. Our dietary preferences aren't as innate as we think they are. They can change.

Habit Reversal without Rules
To break poor eating habits, we must make them into conscious decisions again. It's the opposite process of forming a good habit, which is to make conscious decisions into subconscious non-decisions. Instead of making a decision conscious again, most people go with the dieting strategy and "forbid their habit." Forbidding a core part of your behavioral framework is not smart.

If my rule is that I can't eat ice-cream, that gives me some incentives to eat it. Eating ice-cream would demonstrate my autonomy, show I'm more powerful than the rule, make me feel like I'm in control, and I'd get to eat delicious ice-cream. Sign me up! That's awfully appealing for something that's supposed to dissuade me. Poorly designed rules like this may trigger our desire for control and backfire on us.

Just as processed food becomes more desirable when you forbid it, healthy food struggles with appeal when it becomes the food you "have to eat." It's important to grasp the following concept: People who eat a healthy diet long-term do not need to forbid themselves unhealthy food or force feed themselves healthy food. They just prefer healthy food. This is attainable for you too.

While following the mini habits plan, you can eat cheeseburgers, pizzas, fries, and candy, and drink soda or diet soda. In the meantime, you'll have some mini habits to shift your preferences. To an outsider, it may seem absurd, but that's because we're ignoring superficial change and going for the roots—your habitual dietary preferences.

Once you lose some weight and feel better by eating better food, your perspective of ultra-processed goods will change. As your palate adjusts to the delicious spices and flavors of nutritious food, you'll wonder why you were so focused on *not* eating certain foods in the past when you have

126

so many delicious alternatives to enjoy.

The Pimento Cheese Disaster

I was lying in my bed one night when I suddenly sat up, leaned over the edge of my top bunk, and vomited all over my favorite Detroit Lions pillow below me. You may think I was giving my opinion of their performance on the football field, but no, I was sick with food poisoning. It was the beginning of a miserable couple of days. Earlier that day, I had eaten pimento cheese. It wasn't as fresh as I had hoped.

To this day, I dislike pimento cheese. Before that night, I didn't think pimento cheese was the greatest food ever, but I liked it. The pimento cheese incident changed my preference because of the power of *association*. I associate pimento cheese with food poisoning. Other factors that can affect our food preferences include: texture, appearance, smell, memories, beliefs, health impact, energy impact, gastrointestinal impact (beans, anyone?), and social influence (a common driver of alcohol consumption). Our food preferences involve many more factors than just taste.

Are Preferences Innate or Learned?

Much of the world is at least semi-addicted to salt. Processed and restaurant food comes loaded with salt, and some people still pour extra salt *on top of that*. Is this salt affinity an innate desire? Of course not. We don't need that much salt to live and we're not born loving it—we're taught to like it.

Study: "Newborn infants generally display an aversion or indifference to moderate levels of salt, and it is not until age 2-3 that they prefer salty tastes. Similar effects are observed in low salt intake groups following initial experience with high salt diets, suggesting that at any point during the lifespan the introduction of a high salt diet induces an initial aversion and thereafter requires a period of habituation."[136]

This is bigger than salt. We perform the behaviors that bring us rewards, and from a young age, society trains us to enjoy the foods that cause obesity—high salt, high fat, high sugar foods. Salt, fat, and sugar aren't unhealthy naturally; they're unhealthy in unnatural states and amounts. If you eat a processed food, it's nearly guaranteed to have unnecessary amounts of salt, sugar, and/or fat. At first, we're likely to find this somewhat repulsive. Have you ever tasted something too sweet, too salty, or too rich? If you ate it frequently enough, it would become normal to you.

We've become habituated to eating foods that overdo everything. Flavors, sugars, salt, and fats burst forth from these lab concoctions onto our tongues and overstimulate us. Sensory overstimulation has become not only acceptable, but an *expected* part of eating.

How to Change Your Food Preferences
The following is just my anecdotal experience, and it's probably not the same as your experience, but I'm *not* unique in the fact that my dietary preferences can change.

I had a legendary sweet tooth. I liked sweet food so much that I'd eat non-food items if they were sweet. I vividly remember my sister yelling, "Mom! Stephen ate my Mini Mouse chapstick again!" That was my favorite flavor. I'd also take Tums, gummy vitamins, and candy I snagged from the grocery store into my room. I'd crawl under my bed and eat my forbidden treasures sneakily. (I don't know how I survived childhood.)

I used to love candy and hate kale. Now I dislike candy and enjoy kale. I used to hate sauerkraut. Now I enjoy it. I used to eat at the worst fast food restaurants. Now I never do. I used to drink soda with meals. Now I always drink water.

Food preferences can and will change if there's a reason for change combined with the right approach. I have a healthy diet now, and I'm the guy with weak willpower who loved candy.

You're going to find that, with the complete freedom to eat unhealthy food, it's going to lose a lot of its power over you. Guilt and shame compel us to self-destruct, and when you remove them by making all food fair game, you can make better decisions. By combining this approach with daily mini habits and situational strategies, weight-gaining foods will look differently to you than they ever have before.

I still eat unhealthy foods, but infrequently and in small amounts. When you regain your sensitivity for sugar, salt, and the like, it will take much less of it to satisfy you. I used to pile several scoops of ice-cream into a large cup because bowls couldn't hold enough. Now I rarely eat ice-cream, but when I do, one scoop satisfies me. I never deprive myself. My tastes have just naturally changed, not by banning ice-cream, but by increasing my consumption of healthy food. Once I realized I liked frozen fruit with cinnamon and peanut butter nearly as much as ice-cream, I stopped buying ice-cream.

The Belief and Experience Paradox

If someone must experience change to believe it's possible, but won't try to change if they don't yet believe it's possible, how can they change? Once you're inside this circle, positive change and belief (self-efficacy) will feed each other. But which comes first, belief or change? Or rather, which one is the better foundation?

Start the change, and belief will follow. Mini habits can enact real change, even with little or no belief, because they begin the change and *make you believe*.

It wasn't until my one push-up mini habit morphed into a consistent gym habit that I actually believed I could build meaningful amounts of muscle. After *dabbling* in weight lifting off and on for 3-5 years and seeing nearly nonexistent results, how could I believe? Likewise, how can you believe changing your eating habits will change your weight after dabbling in healthy eating for years and seeing no difference? It takes more than dabbling to see the true effect of a new course of action.

The one perceived benefit of a crash diet or cleanse is that rapid weight results can spark belief, but getting rapid results without sustainability is harmful in the long run to your metabolism and your belief that you can change. Why? This "benefit" turns into a downside once you start eating normally again and regain the (mostly water) weight—you'll go right back to thinking that real change isn't possible. And ironically, you'll think, "If this sudden massive change wasn't enough, then there's no hope." Your problem was that you attempted a massive change—*the brain and body don't like that.* The brain and body like seamless, easy changes, so let's start there.

Make It Easy

The significant advantage that processed foods have always had over healthy foods is their convenience. A bag of chips can sit on your shelf for months, and it is ready to eat the instant you want it. That's easy. Cutting a piece of fruit—one of the easier preparations of healthy food —is comparably difficult.

A healthy meal could mean two hours or more of cooking and cleaning, and if you don't cook the ingredients in time, they may spoil! But there are many ways to make healthy eating as easy (or almost as easy) as eating processed food.

I'm both a bona-fide "health nut" and certified lazy person. This is tricky, because healthy living is generally difficult to do in the USA. This conundrum has forced me to be creative. With these two traits, I've had to learn how to make healthy living *really easy*, or else I'd self-destruct from frustration. Here are some practical ways to make the right choices competitive with the typically easier weight-gaining choices.

Make it Easy Meal Ideas

Buy a rotisserie chicken and use the meat in various dishes through the rest of the week. Rotisserie chickens will last at least 3-4 days in the refrigerator. If you have a family to feed, you'll go through one in no time.

Buy frozen vegetables that you can microwave or cook on the stovetop quickly. Frozen food in general is fantastic, because it retains all of the nutritional value of fresh produce, it doesn't go bad for a very, very long time, and it's easy to prepare.

Master the stir-fry! I favor broccoli, so I'll cook the (frozen) broccoli in a pan with coconut or olive oil, add multi-purpose seasoning (without salt), pepper, ginger, and turmeric, and when it's nearing completion, I toss in some of the pre-cooked chicken to warm it up. It's a healthy and satiating meal. It's easy, it's delicious, and it's fast (maybe 10-20 minutes to prepare). Finding simple healthy routines like this is essential for weight loss, and it's something you'll want to think about a lot, because it makes a big difference. Here are a few more tips.

Learn some slow cooker recipes. Throw it all in the pot and come back when it's ready.

My breakfast is often eggs, cheese, bread, and avocado. Eggs are very easy to prepare for breakfast. If you're really in a hurry, you can microwave them in one minute.[137] There are a number of microwave cookers specially designed for eggs. I have the Nordic Ware Microwave Egg Boiler; it boils four eggs in eight minutes and the shells come off easily. These days, I cook eggs in a pan (olive oil) because it's fast, easy, and tastes better.

Dessert? Frozen fruit is one of the single greatest weight loss inventions in history. It may sound ridiculous, but having to cut fruit is enough resistance for many people (like me) to not eat it. Frozen fruit is already cut and ready to eat. Whenever I want a sweet snack, I'm happy, because my freezer is fully stocked with a variety of frozen fruits. These are good enough to eat right out of the bag, but you can also combine them with whole plain yogurt (which makes for an excellent breakfast, snack, or dessert).

My go-to dessert is a bowl of frozen fruit (usually mangoes, strawberries, and blueberries) with a generous amount of cinnamon on top. It tastes as good as any dessert I've had, and it's *extremely* healthy and weight loss-friendly. When the fruit thaws about halfway, it tastes glorious, and don't forget that fruit is one of the best foods for weight loss (according to both theoretical and observational science).

This is just what I do to make healthy eating easy. There are thousands of other ideas to make food healthier, easier to prepare, and more delicious than you thought possible. But you must look for them. When I wanted to have healthier breakfasts, I researched the easiest ways to prepare eggs. When I wanted to cook more meals at home, I researched and found that cooking meat and veggies in a pan is fast and easy. Whatever your needs, there is certainly an easy solution out there.

Before I cooked my own food, I always assumed it was difficult and took a long time. I've since discovered that it can be quick and easy. If you're averse to cooking, start with the easiest dishes like the ones I've mentioned here, and see if it's as bad as you thought. If you still think cooking is the worst thing in the world, then consider a healthy meal delivery service. You can get home-cooked, healthy meals delivered to you in more places than ever. Most of them cater to health-conscious individuals, so you won't get a lot of the fattening additives that restaurants use.

Instant, Permanent, Easy Substitutions
There are a few easy substitutions that everyone can make immediately for long-lasting benefits. These substitutions can take you far all on their own and they don't "cost" you anything. You make the decision once and live life as usual.

Switch to whole grain products. It's astonishing how much better whole grains are for you than refined grains. It's not "a little bit better." Whole grains are a quality food, and refined grains are weight-gaining. Whole grains have more antioxidants, fiber, and nutrients, and are slower to digest. If you don't think they taste as good as their refined counterparts (like white rice and white flour), you can *learn* to enjoy them as much or more. Tip: Think about the health benefits of the food as you eat it. I believe this is what changed my mind about sauerkraut and kale.

Exclusively use coconut oil and olive oil for cooking. You know that one oil you always cook with? Coconut oil and olive oil are better for your health and your waistline. They have great flavor, too!

Use olive oil, herbs, spices, and vinegar for dressings and dips. We want things to taste good, but that doesn't mean we have to gain weight with the standard "soybean oil and sugar" dressings sold in grocery stores. Olive oil and balsamic vinegar make for a great salad dressing. You can also add black pepper, herbs, cheese, and spices to flavor salads. If you're having (whole grain) garlic bread, olive oil and fresh garlic will make you dance.

Need dip? Go for hummus and guacamole! Ranch dressing is soybean oil with make-up on. Instead, use hummus or guacamole for a veggie dip. Healthy hummus and guacamole can be prepared and even store-bought (read the ingredients!).

Use large forks and small plates. If you want to change your dinnerware to psychologically help with portion control, the right combination is small plates and large forks, which have both been shown in studies to lead to less food consumption. It's worth mentioning because it's a one-time change that could help, but mindful eating is more important. You can do well, even if you're unfortunate enough to have small forks and large plates.

Since portion size is less important than eating quality food, it's probably not worth throwing out all of your dishes in favor of a smaller set. Rather, simply be aware that plate and bowl size affects your portion choices, and adjust accordingly. But try to pick enough food. One study showed that people ate less when they "filled their plate" with enough food, instead of going back for seconds.

Whatever you do, try not to let *plate size* determine your satiety. Believe your body when it tells you it's had enough, regardless of how much food remains on the plate. Buy some Tupperware and practice saving food for later when you're satisfied. It'll be there when you're hungry again.

Eating Psychology

Never require yourself to finish or "clean" your plate. It would be interesting to know the statistics on how many people eat with the goal to finish all of the food. Logically, using the amount of food that's on your plate to determine how much you eat doesn't make any sense, especially at restaurants, since *they* determine your serving size.

Think about two opposing eating habits: When you're served a plate of food, one possible habit is to attempt to eat everything on it. Another possible habit is to disregard the serving size and eat the precise amount your body tells you to eat, no more and no less. If you have the plate-finishing habit, that means you have been ignoring your body's signals. Put another way, it means you're probably way out of sync with your body's satiety signaling. If you ignore what your body is telling you in favor of the almighty "finish the plate" goal, that's exactly the behavior you'll get good at. The good news is that your body still sends these signals; you just have to decide to pay closer attention.

Finishing the food on your plate is less important than your health and well-being. Wouldn't you agree? To clarify, this isn't about eating fewer calories. Healthy people aim for neither calorie restriction nor calorie surplus.

Successful weight loss requires no counting, monitoring, or micromanagement of portion sizes. All it requires is that you eat mindfully. Mindful eaters never aim to finish their plate, because their decision is internally based. They may or may not end up finishing, but it has nothing to do with the amount of food on their plate and everything to do with what their body is telling them.

As for when to stop eating, eat to satisfaction, not to explosion. Overeating is a cultural and habitual practice. In Japan, there's a popular concept called "hara hachi bu," which basically means "eat to 80% fullness." This is a solid guideline, and it isn't semi-starvation. When you stop at 80% fullness, you'll enjoy the whole eating experience more. Inflammation and hormonal issues can disrupt the way your satiety signaling operates, but this is best treated by mindfully eating healthy foods as a staple.

Alcohol Strategy

A great strategy for alcohol consumption is to simultaneously drink water. If you have several drinks in a night for fun, I'm not going to stop you, and you might not stop yourself, so instead of counting the night as a loss, make an effort to drink water too. This will help keep you hydrated, prevent hangovers, and minimize the damage of drinking too much alcohol.

One of the biggest risks for alcohol is how it might impact your food eating habits. It lowers inhibition and may increase your appetite for weight-gaining foods. I recommend looking at your previous behavior to form your strategy.

If you find yourself overdoing alcohol whenever you begin drinking, try to drink less often, to minimize your alcohol-related weight gain. If you always stop at one or two drinks, then you're probably fine, unless drinking causes poor eating habits, in which case you can either try to reroute your habits (with the temptation strategy we'll cover later) or drink on fewer nights.

Food Mini Habit Ideas

The preceding information is something to keep in mind, but not a "mandatory" part of this strategy. The following mini habit ideas will be the foundation of your successful change into a healthier person.

When you're down, sick, or have low energy, your mini habits are easy enough to accomplish. When you're full of energy and motivation to change, you'll have bonus activities to further your progress. You'll act more consistently and intelligently than you ever have before, because *your goal will finally be adaptable to you*, allowing you to achieve precisely what you are able to each day. Unlike most strategies, which require a superhuman amount of willpower for consistent success, this strategy is built for success, no matter what state you're currently (or will be) in.

The Ideal Mini Habit
The ideal mini habit is something extremely easy to do that also begins the process of engagement. For example, one push-up can begin the process of exercising. Eating one raw vegetable can begin the process of eating more vegetables. When you begin a process, you're likely to continue doing it. Put another way, you're most likely to do what you just did.

Whether or not you do bonus reps is optional, so don't feel bad if you don't. If you *never* do extra for a full month, then ask yourself if your mini habit really starts the process, or if you need to add in one more step to get engaged with the behavior. Mini habits are sparks. Any spark has the potential to become an inferno.

If you can achieve more on any day, do it. It feels great to *overachieve* goals, even small ones. We're used to setting high targets, falling short of them, and feeling inadequate when we do. This time, you'll meet or exceed your goals every day. Think about the psychological difference: A modest "normal goal" is to run a mile every day. A typical mini habit is to run for 30 seconds. If you run for half a mile, according to the normal goal, you've failed. According to the mini habit, you've not only succeeded—you've done more than expected!

A mini habit encourages progress in any amount. A typical goal suggests that progress is only valuable in large chunks, which is so inaccurate and nonsensical that it makes me angry. Every single thing on planet Earth is comprised of infinitesimally small matter. Every single success can be traced back to small individual steps, so this is a way to align your intentions with the way progress and success naturally work. The only kind of big "chunk wins" possible in life are things like winning the lottery (good luck). All of life's other wins—such as achieving goals and losing weight—are based on your small daily decisions and actions.

It feels *good* to win, and when you start to win every day, you will change into a winner. Yeah, it sounds cheesy to say that, but those who win frequently act more confidently and proactively because they learn to expect success, and their success will fuel further success. I call it success cycling.

Many people try to turn motivation into success, but they have it backwards. Success and motivation fuel each other, but the most reliable *starting point* is success, which leads to motivation, which then leads to more success. The mini habits on this page give you an opportunity for daily success, no matter how unmotivated you may feel. When you string together days, weeks, and months of this success, you're going to become a better, stronger, more successful version of your current self. The experience is difficult to put into words, because at no point does it seem reasonable that such small behaviors could do so much for one's life. But they do, and it's thrilling.

Food Mini Habits

My only fear is that you'll be disappointed by this list, as it's quite short and the behaviors are simple. This is a good thing, but it might not feel that way if you're accustomed to highly demanding, complex weight loss systems that dieting culture has created. This is different, because those don't work! The strongest strategies are as simple as possible while still being effective.

Within each of these ideas is a massive amount of variation, so you won't ever be short for options. But the basic ideas are simple because weight loss is accomplished by increased mindfulness, a healthier diet, and increased movement. The way you eat food, your emotional health, and your perspective can also impact your weight (mostly by indirectly affecting those core three factors), so there will be some mini habits related to those.

As you look through these and think about which ones you'd like to try, don't think about doing them all. You want to have a *maximum* of four mini habits, such as two food mini habits and one or two fitness mini habits. In chapter eight, we'll discuss exactly how to integrate these ideas (and the general and fitness mini habits) into your life with a mini habit plan.

Eat one extra serving of fruit: It's important to know how much one serving is so you know what to aim for. One serving of fruit is one apple, one large cup of berries, one banana, or one orange. It's also important to always have fruit on hand if this is your mini habit. If you like it as easy as possible like me, buy frozen fruit, as it's ready to eat and doesn't spoil. I strongly recommend buying organic berries and peaches, as the conventional ones contain a high amount of pesticides. Berries and peaches are part of the "dirty dozen" (a name for the most pesticide-laden foods). If you buy conventional, rinse well.

Fruit Bonus: Eat additional fruit or add full-fat plain yogurt to your fruit.

Eat one extra serving of fresh vegetables: For some people, aiming to consume one serving of vegetables doesn't make sense, since they already consume that daily. In that case, you can get more specific, like one serving of raw vegetables or one more serving than is typical. Ideas include: one full carrot, three pieces of broccoli, two pieces of cauliflower, half a bell pepper (red, green, yellow), one celery stick, one fourth of a cucumber, one handful of spinach, eight slices of raw radish, or whatever suits your tastes. If you want, you can count fruits that seem like vegetables as vegetables (e.g., four cherry tomatoes or half an avocado).

If you want dip for your raw vegetables, use hummus, which, in its simplest form, is pureed chickpeas, olive oil, lemon juice, tahini (ground sesame seeds), garlic, salt, and pepper. Another option is guacamole, which is avocado, onions, garlic, tomato, lime, salt, and pepper. Be cautious about buying prepackaged dips from the store, as you may end up getting three bathtubs of salt in every serving, added preservatives (inflammatory), and even sugar. "Vegetable dips" are almost always disguised soybean oil. Eating vegetables covered in soybean oil and other weight-gaining ingredients is not ideal. It may be a stepping stone to the ideal (if that's the only way you'll eat them, do it), but it's not the ideal.

Vegetable Bonus: Eat additional vegetables or go all in with a mega salad!

Make one mini healthy food upgrade: This is a vague mini habit, but in practice, that can be a good thing. Make one small healthy upgrade per day or at mealtime (depending on your plan and cue). Maybe you're at a restaurant and you swap your typical side of fries for a baked potato, green beans, or a salad. Upgrade! Maybe you're at home ready to snack it up, and you think to eat chips, but decide to eat some unsalted raw nuts first. Upgrade! Maybe you go for the Cobb salad over lasagna, and you ask the waiter for olive oil and vinegar instead of the usual soybean oil dressing variants. Double upgrade! Every day is full of food decisions, and you don't need to overhaul them all at once (nor should you try). This strategy cements that correct perspective in your mind by asking you to make one small upgrade of your choosing.

Here's the opposite of an upgrade: skipping meals and not eating when you're hungry. The next time you think to make yourself hungry as a way to lose weight, read the introduction of this book again. It will remind you that artificially restricting calories is a weight-gaining move. If it's 11 PM and you're usually hungry at this time, but aren't feeling hungry on a particular day, then no, you don't need to eat. Listen to your body. Eat when you're hungry, don't when you're not, and use mini habits to shift *how* you eat.

Food Upgrade Bonus: Double or triple your upgrade. There's no upper limit!

Prepare one healthy meal at home: This mini habit is completely dependent on your current situation and habits. Some people always cook at least one meal per day, while others eat out all the time. I suggest breakfast, because it's very easy to make a healthy breakfast. (Eggs are great for weight loss because they are nutritious and make you feel full.[138] Fruit and yogurt are a fine option as well. Add cinnamon!) For many people, this mini habit will be too big to start out with. It depends on your current habits. If you can't do it every day, don't try to do it every day. Either choose a different mini habit or aim for five days per week or something like that. Daily mini habits are best for a few reasons (consistency, daily mindfulness, time to habit, etc.), but again, it's important to make this work for your lifestyle.

Don't cheat yourself: Most microwave meals aren't healthy. Cereal and grilled cheese are not weight loss weapons. White pasta and marinara sauce is a weight-gainer (whole wheat pasta and olive oil, though, is a decent choice).

Healthy Meal Upgrade: Prepare another meal, or make enough for healthy leftovers!

Drink one glass of water: Water is a weight loss WEAPON for the reasons we covered earlier. You might think it's a bad idea to aim for one glass of water per day, because we're supposed to drink more than that. But pay attention to that thought, because that's *exactly* the type of thought we want to be having! Now you're mindful of how much water you're drinking per day, and thinking "I can do more than one per day," instead of feeling overwhelmed by "having to drink 8 glasses per day." Drinking one glass won't ever prevent you from drinking another; it will only make you more likely to do so. Remember, the strategy is not the same as the end goal.

Too boring? I like the taste of plain water, but some people like some zing in their drink, and that's okay. Nature has multiple answers. If you are accustomed to flavored beverages, you can make your transition away from "the dark side" easier by spicing your water up with fruits, spices, and carbonation. Lemons, limes, mint, apples, cinnamon, mango, ginger, cucumber, strawberries, oranges, and basically any other fruit (especially citrus) can liven up your water in a healthy way. Lemon is one of the most popular healthy water additives for good reason. It's tasty, it's packed with flavonoids and antioxidants (like Vitamin C), and it won't take much of it to add flavor.

If this is really important to you (if you drink a lot of sodas, lattes, and the like, then flavoring your water could be crucial to your success), you can buy a water infuser pitcher and you'll have delicious tasting water ready all day long. You'll find plenty of infuser options on Amazon.[139] Just throw your fruits, vegetables, and spices into the infuser with some water and put it in the fridge. Don't forget the cinnamon! Please, never forget cinnamon. (If you have some cinnamon nearby, go over there and smell it. It's my favorite smell. My family had a cat named Cinnamon, and, as a kid, I used to sing to her. She'd flatten her ears out of love.)

Like most unhealthy foods and drinks, soda's main advantage is availability. If you infused water with your favorite fruits and spices and always had that available, I bet you could easily move on from cheap syrupy soda. Soda tastes great, but why drink it when you can get delicious beverages without the downsides?

Perhaps you don't want to go through the trouble of infusing your water with fruits and spices when there are so many ready-made drinks out there. I understand. A very easy and effective alternative is to buy 100% fruit juice, but instead of drinking it straight, add just a little bit of it to a full glass of water to flavor it. You'll be surprised how refreshing this is, and you won't be getting an overdose of fructose from drinking 100% fruit juice.

All fruit juices (even 100% fruit juice) are weight-gaining beverages in anything but small quantities. Fruits are one of the best foods for weight loss in their whole form, but they become weight-gaining as juices. Just add enough to flavor your water to satisfaction.

Avoid packets of powder for flavor. They all contain sweeteners. I've never seen a good one. They can be a decent exercise drink, but not for general drinking.

Water Bonus: Two, three, four glasses of water? Oh, you're good.

Chew each bite 30+ times: This is per bite, not per mouthful. This practice has multiple benefits: You'll digest your food easily. You'll taste and enjoy your meal more. You'll automatically eat more mindfully. You'll be nearly guaranteed to eat less because your "I'm full" response will have enough time to register. Set a "chew count" per bite and practice it. Eventually, it will become habitual, just as your current chewing count is habitual.

I've tested out the 30 chews per bite mini habit and it's great. Digestion is much better, the food is more enjoyable, and it's tougher to overeat. I did find some issues with the flat 30 chews per bite rule. In practice, I would adjust to 15+ bites for softer foods like fruit and 45+ for tougher foods like meat, and I think that's a good general guideline to follow.

Chewing your food well reduces food consumption for the same satiety and greater satisfaction. That's a huge, irreplaceable win. A Chinese study found that men of all weights ate about 12% fewer calories when they chewed their food more. Scientifically speaking, they found more chewing resulted in decreased ghrelin levels (the hunger hormone). When left to their natural chewing preferences, the obese men ate more quickly and chewed fewer times. How many more chews did it take to decrease calorie consumption by 12%? 25 more. They started with about 15 chews, and were then instructed to chew 40 times, which resulted in the change.[140] In my testing, I found 40 chews to be a bit excessive, and, if it's a chore to do it, you probably won't. I find that it works best to require less and encourage bonus chews. That said, if you want to and can chew 40 times, go for it. You can't overchew food; you can only underchew it.

Chewing Bonus: On any bite, go for more chews. Can you do 50? At higher chew counts, it becomes surprisingly difficult to not swallow your food.

7

Fitness Strategy

Let's Make it Fun

"Fitness needs to be perceived as fun and games or we subconsciously avoid it."
~ Alan Thicke

Mindset

Many overweight people associate exercise with strenuous activity, severe discomfort, and even pain. They think they have to "punish" themselves and their body in order to get the significant fat loss they want. Extreme workouts can definitely bring results, but if the experience worsens your relationship with exercise, those results won't last.

A study found that those who had internalized the stigma of being overweight had lower self-esteem and avoided exercise.[141] This seems paradoxical if you think in terms of simple cause and effect. If a person wants to lose weight, and exercise helps weight loss, why would they avoid exercise? Because they find it uncomfortable. Because they're overwhelmed by society's pressure to be thin. Because they think they have to climb 15 mountains before exercise will "show a benefit." Because they focus on the stigma of being overweight. In summary, it's because they have the wrong perspective and the wrong relationship with exercise, which makes them not even want to *think* about it, let alone do it.

What's more valuable: losing 15 pounds in one month from strenuous exercise you hate or losing no weight in a month but enjoying exercise more than when you started? I hope you said the latter, because it is roughly 198 times superior than any exercise program ever devised. You may question it, because 15 pounds is a good amount of weight, but the return from a healthier relationship with exercise—and the knowledge of how to improve it further—will continue to pay off for *the rest of your life*. Choosing the 15 pounds in one month would be like taking a one-time payment of $200 now instead of receiving $100 a week for the rest of your life.

Imagine the following. What if you *enjoyed* exercise? What if you smiled when you thought of it? What if you did it because you wanted to do it, not because you wanted a result from it or felt pressured or shamed into it? This concept is foreign to many people, because exercise is portrayed everywhere as "the way to a flatter stomach" and "the fast track to burning calories and losing weight." If that's all exercise is to you now, you're going to be very excited to find it's much more than that.

In keeping with our theme, we're going to focus on our long-term relationship with exercise, rather than on using it to get a short-term result. I've done this to transform multiple areas of my life with mini habits. One of those areas was reading. There was a time when reading was a chore I only did when I wanted a specific result from it. Reading to me was like exercise to most people trying to lose weight. Here's the story.

How I Repaired My Relationship with Reading

When I was younger, I enjoyed reading books, especially the *Goosebumps* and *Choose Your Own Adventure* series. Then school happened. Some youth rebel with sex, drugs, and alcohol. I rebelled against homework. Aren't I wild? I know most kids don't like homework, but I *despised it*. I had to spend eight hours a day at school five days a week, and then they tried to take even more of my freedom by giving me busywork at home! No way!

A big portion of my homework was assigned reading. The more I was forced to read for school, the more I resisted. I was rebellious, sure, but this evolved beyond *mere* rebellion. My relationship with reading had changed. It was no longer a fascinating adventure into a fictional world or an enlightening nonfiction discovery, it became a dull "do it or suffer the consequences" activity. In my own time, I stopped reading for fun.

In college, I was excited to see a British Literature class available in which we would read and discuss books by two of my favorite authors, J. R. R. Tolkien and C. S. Lewis. *I didn't read a single assigned book that semester.*

My subconscious wanted freedom, but from what? Reading was not actually the enemy; it just seemed like it, because it was the tool used to take my freedom away. I only wanted my freedom back. Does that sound familiar to your experience with exercise? If you regularly feel overwhelming pressure to exercise, then you have a broken relationship with it. Society and weight loss books and programs tend to turn exercise from "just moving and using your body" into a resentment-ridden job.

My third ever mini habit was to read two pages in a book per day. It was easy, lightweight, and changed my relationship with reading over time. I read roughly one book a month these days. It's nothing amazing, I know, but it is *relatively amazing* considering I used to read, at most, one book per year. I've even read thousands of studies researching for my books, because I can do it on my terms. I can do it from a place of freedom.

Within that story is precisely the difference between this book and every other "dieting" book you've read. I'm not prescribing you an exercise routine to "torch" calories or "shred your abs." I'm asking you to work on your *relationship* with exercise (and food, too), because, if you can change that, *you* will drive your own results for life. Self-generated results sure beat a 30-day program that leaves you wondering what to do on day 31.

As you read through the suggested types of exercise for weight loss later in this chapter, keep in mind that exercise type is less important than repairing the damage done by seeing it as a job, as punishment for being overweight, or whatever other kind of dysfunctional relationship you may have formed with it.

What is to dislike about exercise, after all? We move every day, and that is exercise. If you dislike exercise, it's probably the same situation as me and reading, and the solution is to get to know it again without all the baggage.

After exercising in the past, have you noticed that you feel better about yourself? Exercise is intrinsically and biologically rewarding on multiple levels. Other than improving basically every known health marker, it helps you sleep better, improves your sex life, improves your ability to focus, boosts your baseline energy level, feels good (as endorphins are released), *chemically* improves your mood, and is equal to medication in the treatment of depression and anxiety.[142] As some have said before, if exercise were a pill, it would be a blockbuster drug with record-breaking sales.

A long list of exercise benefits is irrelevant if you can't get yourself to do it. Before my one push-up per day mini habit, I failed to go to the gym consistently for 10 years, so I completely understand the frustration of wanting the benefits but not feeling up to the task. Understand that a lack of motivation to exercise is determined by your subconscious mind, and you can change it with an exercise mini habit.

This is critical: the end result is ultimately determined by the goal, but it is not dependent on the goal. The goal matters, but not in the way people think it does. In the push-up story, you might recall that when I aimed for 30 minutes (goal), I got nothing (result). But when I aimed for one push-up (goal), I got 30 minutes (result). The goal and result are nearly opposites, showing the counterintuitive nature of behavior change. The explanation, however, is simple—failure demoralizes us and success motivates us.

If you set a small goal and meet it, you've already succeeded on a small level. You can stack these small wins indefinitely, and you'll end up with a bucket of small wins adding up to a huge win. But if you get greedy, aim for the big win right away, and fail for whatever reason, you'll feel discouraged. In many cases, the initial failure is motivation, which we cannot fully control. It continuously baffles me that this boneheaded strategy is the mainstream way that we're taught to pursue goals. I believe we get "dream big" confused with the strategies needed to reach those dreams. If you want to succeed at something, dream big and take small actions repeatedly (not "dream big" and "take massive action").

A mini habit is a unique challenge in that it's fun(ny). You're going to be thinking, "I can't believe I'm aiming for one push-up a day," or "Walk to the end of my driveway? Am I seriously doing this? I hope my neighbors don't ask me what I'm doing out here." Laughing at your exercise goals is quite a change from the traditional daunting approach.

In addition to your exercise mini habit, you will be encouraged to do "bonus reps," but that's completely up to you. If you do extra, you'll be doing it because you want to do it (autonomy), not because of some arbitrary, controlling rule. The small size of the mini habit means you won't feel controlled by it, and the flexibility for bonus reps will supercharge your sense of autonomy because it's choice-driven instead of goal-driven. You can use whatever momentum, motivation, or willpower you have at your disposal to do additional exercise.

On the days you need a break, you can do your mini habit and walk away with a win. Even the minimum mini habit is a win if done daily because it is enough to change your subconscious feelings about exercise. Not only are you practicing frequent exercise, but you're also practicing the small step habit, or the idea that even a small step forward is useful. This will gradually replace any residual beliefs you may have about exercise being miserable and only useful in large amounts. I hope this makes sense in text form, because in practice it will blow your mind (in time, since we are talking about brain change).

Exercise Vs. Active Living

Most experts speak of how exercise is less important than diet in the weight loss battle, and that's true in the short term. You can't outrun a poor diet. In 30 minutes of running, you can burn about 400 calories (depending on your pace and weight), which only amounts to a single Burger King cheeseburger.

Athletes Michael Phelps (swimming) and J. J. Watt (American football) both train for several hours on some days. They have something else extraordinary in common. Both of these athletes have been said to consume more than 9,000 calories a day while training! Despite eating more than three times as much as a typical person, they don't get fat, because their metabolism burns through those calories like a bonfire burns through Uncle Jesse's marshmallow. If you were to try to calculate the calories burned from their training, you'd get a number well under 9,000 calories, because many of those calories are burned at rest. Metabolism matters more than calories, which is why these guys can eat like horses and not get fatter, while another person starves herself on 800 calories a day and gets fatter soon after, because of increased appetite and decreased metabolism.

Phelps and Watt have a *lifestyle* of training, but the average person needn't adopt such an extreme exercise plan—we can make big strides with incrementally more active lifestyles than we currently have. The lesson isn't that we need to exercise for seven hours a day, it's that our *general lifestyle* determines our metabolism. While it is important to exercise for overall health, it's not as important as being active for weight loss. Today, we seem to think a healthy lifestyle is to remain motionless for 23.5 hours, and then run for 30 minutes on a treadmill. A 30-minute session on the treadmill counts for a lot, but so do the other 23 hours and 30 minutes of the day. According to juststand.org, 86% of Americans sit all day at work. This can easily change.

The Mortality of Sitting
In 2003, 6,329 study participants over the age of six were given an activity monitor. On average, participants wore the monitor for 13.9 hours. Here's what they found: "Overall, participants spent 54.9% of their monitored time, or 7.7 hours/day, in sedentary behaviors."[143] Estimates for daily sitting range from 8 hours to as high as 15 hours for some people.

Studies on prolonged sitting:

- A 2014 study found that prolonged sitting is a major health hazard for older women (93,000 participants).[144]
- A 2010 study found that prolonged sitting increased mortality

146

rates and decreased life spans across the board (120,000+ participants).[145]

- Another study published in 2012 had 222,497 people answer a questionnaire. It also found that "prolonged sitting is a risk factor for all-cause mortality, independent of physical activity."[146]

Basically, studies show that sitting for long periods of time is lethal. But it's also a missed opportunity to lose weight. In 2005, 10 lean and 10 obese volunteers were given underwear that tracked their body position every 0.5 seconds. (Who comes up with these ideas?) The magic underwear data showed that obese people sat two and a half *more* hours per day. Researchers said, "If obese individuals adopted the NEAT-enhanced behaviors of their lean counterparts, they might expend an additional 350 calories (kcal) per day."[147]

The acronym NEAT stands for "non-exercise activity thermogenesis." It represents all of the calorie burning your body does outside of intentional exercise. You are constantly using energy, as it takes energy to breathe, think, move, and circulate blood. How much energy you use outside of exercise is highly variable. Athletes like Michael Phelps and J. J. Watt might burn more calories at rest than some people do while exercising.

I believe that NEAT is an underrated key to weight loss. People are prone to devalue small improvements, such as the calories burned standing as opposed to sitting, but the theme of this book is how small but consistent improvements always create better-than-expected results.

The typical American worker sleeps, wakes up, and immediately begins *resting* in a chair for the entire day. A small change like standing up for part of your work day could make a big difference, not only in your metabolism, but in your productivity.

Dr. John Buckley, a researcher at the University of Chester, put sitting and standing to the test. He found that standing participants' hearts beat at 10 more beats per minute. "That makes a difference of about 0.7 of a calorie per minute,"[148] Buckley says. I did the math, and that is 42 more calories burned per hour, and that's only if you don't dance while standing. If you go beyond standing and lightly exercise on the job, Dr. James Levine says of the various methods of active desk enhancements, "[The obese can] burn about 150 extra calories an hour."[149] The effect is even greater than these calorie numbers, as it will likely improve your baseline metabolism over time (if done consistently).

Sitting isn't *precisely* the problem; it's the fact that most people remain motionless when they sit. There are products out now like the Deskcycle, an exercise bike that fits under your desk so you can pedal while sitting. There's also a stepper you can place under your desk.

A NEAT Idea

Most NEAT activities take up none of your time. These are alternate ways of living that simply involve you using your body rather than relying on machines and chairs. Standing instead of sitting. Stairs instead of the elevator. Walking instead of driving.

The first focal point should be your job lifestyle, as we spend so many of our waking hours at work. As a writer, I spend a majority of the time at my desk, so I use a product called the Varidesk, a platform you put on top of your existing desk that extends to standing height and back down to desk level. It's very fast and easy to lift it into standing mode or put it back into sitting mode. While this product is nice to have, it isn't cheap.

Standing desk solutions don't have to be expensive. When I first wanted to trying standing up to work, I stacked cardboard boxes on top of my desk. (It didn't look stylish, but neither do sweatpants.) It was free and it worked fine. I'd move my laptop up and down to switch between sitting and standing.

Consider buying a stand-up desk, treadmill desk, or creating one yourself. Warning: don't try to stand up the entire work day on day one. You will regret it the next day. Start with an hour or two per day and work your way up to half of the workday. A fatigue mat is very helpful. Talk to your employer; they might be willing to accommodate your needs (it is increasingly common these days, given the startling research on sitting's dangers and the productivity boost gained from standing).

Standing advice: When at a standing desk, don't lock your knees and stand still. Move, dance, shift, and change it up. Standing in the same spot for a long time is better than sitting, but it's not great if you don't move at all. (This can also be made into a mini habit, as you'll see at the end of this chapter.)

One of the greatest benefits of a standing desk is how easy it is to walk away from it and come back. If you work in a creative field, then you know the difficulty of creating things. The answers don't always just "come to you." Sometimes you need to take a step back. At a standing desk, you can literally do that. I can't tell you how powerful this subtle freedom has been. While sitting, you could conceivably do the same, but the small extra amount of resistance from having to get up is enough to keep us in our seat on more occasions.

When using a standing desk, I've had more energy, my mental sharpness has increased, and my productivity has been effortless at times (something I hadn't experienced before). Increased productivity while standing is counterintuitive in a way, because standing uses more energy, theoretically leaving less energy for the brain to use. But the way our bodies work is quite different than that surface-level idea. Sitting slows metabolism and standing stokes it. Higher metabolism means higher energy, which is why I'm dancing as I'm typing this. Light activity doesn't wear us down as much as it jumpstarts all of our systems. For this reason, walkers and joggers often remark that some of their best ideas come during their workouts. If you're all-out sprinting, then you won't be able to think about much else, because your body is putting all of its resources toward that action.

When I sit down to work, I feel lazier and waste more time. Sometimes I'll fall asleep in my chair. Sedentary behavior generates sedentary behavior! While standing, I've found my motivation and energy to work are at least double what they are while sitting.

If you've explored all avenues and it's somehow still not possible for you to stand up sometimes at work, set an alarm or chime to go off every hour or half hour, and then get up and move around when it goes off. You can do jumping jacks, push-ups, pace, or even perform a quick jig for the pleasure of anyone nearby. Just a few seconds is enough to awaken your sleepy metabolism from its resting state. While this is simple and easy to do, the impact will not be inconsequential.

However you accomplish it, the goal is to get to a situation in which you aren't motionless for most of your day. Make it a priority, because it's important for your health and may help you lose weight. One of the key ways I stay active in my sedentary occupation is my penchant for listening to music throughout the day and dancing to it often.

In the next section, I'll give you additional (but optional) "mini challenges" if you want to increase your NEAT and raise your resting metabolism. This is the introduction to the strategy we want to pursue. We want to move, and not just while we're working out, and not in the high-pressure way that weight loss programs prescribe (because that makes people hate being active).

Exercise Type

After I moved to Seattle, for the first time in my life, I gained a noticeable amount of fat in my abdominal and love handle area. (Getting fatter while writing a weight loss book was not the plan.) I thought the fat gain was especially odd, as I had been going to the gym more than ever before in my life since moving here! I was, however, trying to eat a lot to gain muscle mass. In addition to eating more, I had stopped playing basketball regularly for the first time in as long as I can remember.

Since I already had an exercise habit in place and I wanted to decrease my body fat, I asked the question that everyone asks when attempting to lose fat: What type of exercise should I do? Should I focus on endurance, continue to lift weights, or go for high-intensity interval training (referred to as HIIT from this point forward)?

Not all exercise is equal for weight loss, and the most popular type might be the least effective. When beginning a new weight loss plan, what do most people do first? They get on the treadmill for endurance training. This sort of moderate exercise has shown to be an inferior way to trigger fat loss.

The Science on Exercising for Weight Loss
A 1989 study looked at the body composition of 18 men and 9 women after training for 18 months to run a marathon. At the end of one year, the men saw a modest 2.4 kg decrease in body fat, but the women were unchanged. Can you imagine running for a year and a half without any fat loss? It wouldn't be very encouraging!

Exercise physiologist Mary Kennedy ran a pilot study consisting of 64 marathoners, comparing their weight before and after training. Their training was three months of running four days per week. About 11% gained weight, 11% lost weight, and 78% stayed the same.[150] This suggests their marathon training had no effect on body weight.

Did these people waste their time? Absolutely not. The benefits of exercise extend far beyond fat loss. But if fat loss is your goal, there are better-suited types of exercise than running at moderate speed on the human version of a hamster wheel.

Research shows that HIIT exercise is the best form of exercise for burning off fat, especially in the abdominal area. So perhaps my problem was that I stopped playing basketball. Full court basketball is similar to HIIT, with its alternating periods of sprinting and active rest.

As a general rule, if you can handle high-intensity exercise—almost every person can handle some form of it—choose that over moderate-intensity cardio. Studies show that high-intensity exercise is very effective for fat loss, especially around the abdomen.[151]

When a 15-week HIIT program was compared to a 20-week endurance training (ET) program, they found that "the HIIT program induced a more pronounced reduction in subcutaneous adiposity compared with the ET program."[152] The difference was enormous: "The decrease in the sum of six subcutaneous skinfolds induced by the HIIT program was ninefold greater than by the ET program." If you could get nine times the results in less time, and with less energy expenditure, would you? For less than half the amount of megajoules (an energy measurement unit) expended, HIIT produced nine times the fat loss.[153] This means that, for the same amount of energy expended, HIIT was actually 18 times more effective than ET at decreasing fat. Wow.

Another study divided 45 women into three groups: steady state, high intensity, and a control group. Both exercise groups improved their cardiovascular fitness level. "However, only the HIIE [high-intensity intermittent exercise] group had a significant reduction in total body mass (TBM), fat mass (FM), trunk fat and fasting plasma insulin levels."[154]

Not convinced yet? (I am.) This next study is the most shocking. Ten men and ten women were split into two groups. One group ran 30-60 minutes on the treadmill three times per week. Another group ran four to six 30-second sprints (that's only two to three minutes of exercise time) with four minutes of recovery time between sprints, and they also did it three times per week. Fat mass decreased 5.8% in the endurance training group, but in the sprint interval group, fat mass decreased a whopping 12.4%![155] That's more than twice as much, and in far less time spent exercising. If that's not enough good news for HIIT, another small study found that intense interval training *reduced the appetite* of male participants.[156] (See the footnote for more details.)[157]

Lastly, Google "sprinter body vs. marathon body." Look at the difference in body type between these athletes. Sprinters, male and female, generally have much greater muscle mass than marathoners, who sometimes look emaciated and frail. Brief high-intensity exercise torches body fat without taking your lean muscle with it.

Personally, if I'm going to be pounding my joints for miles at a time, there had better be a payoff. Basketball isn't easy on the joints, but I love to play it and it keeps me fit. Marathons aren't fun to most people, and, if you don't enjoy them, they aren't worth it. Some studies have even found negative cardiac implications from endurance training,[158] including heart scarring.[159] For example, a study found that 50% of a group of 12 lifetime marathoners showed signs of heart scarring, while none of the age-matched control group did.[160] This is not definite proof that endurance training is harmful. For example, the heart scarring study was about *lifetime marathoners*, which most of us are not. I do think it's a good example of how endurance training in extreme amounts wears down the body, rather than making it stronger.

It's common to assume that time is the most important factor in exercise, but all these studies show that *intensity* matters a lot more than time does, and that recovery time is a smart idea. This happens to be a very mini habit-friendly data point, as we're aiming for activities that initially only require small amounts of our time. Intense activity is somewhat intimidating to someone not accustomed to it, but much less so when it's for seconds.

Before we get into high-intensity training considerations, there is a very important caveat to this information. High-intensity exercise is not the best form of exercise. *The best form of exercise is the type you'll actually do.* You may have heard this before, and it's true. I believe most people will prefer high-intensity exercise because it takes less time and gives much better results, but if you will only run for 30 minutes on the treadmill while watching your favorite TV show, then you should absolutely do that. Exercise of any kind will help your health and possibly your weight. If you want to try high-intensity exercise, here are some considerations.

High-Intensity Training Considerations
1. Consider the safety of high-intensity exercise. I'll try not to

sound like a pharmaceutical commercial, but talk to your doctor about high-intensity exercise, especially if you have any doubts or pre-existing health problems. If you are able to do it, intense exercise has been found to produce greater cardiovascular capacity and cardioprotective benefits than moderate exercise, but it "could acutely and transiently increase the risk of sudden cardiac death and myocardial infarction in susceptible persons."[161] Here's some data on that last point to ease your concerns.

A study tracked 4,846 coronary heart disease patients performing all types of exercise. In 129,456 hours of moderate exercise, there was one instance of exercise-induced cardiac arrest. In 46,364 hours of intense exercise, there were two instances of exercise-induced cardiac arrest. You can see that both rates of occurrence are extremely low, but higher with more intense exercise. These incidence rates were low even with heart disease patients, who are at the highest risk for a cardiac event. Since higher-intensity exercise produces greater benefits for heart health and weight loss, and cardiac events are rare even in heart disease patients, it's almost always the better choice.

2. The primary benefit of exercising is not to get a fat loss result. Fat loss is a side effect of living healthier. The whole reason fat loss makes us look more attractive is because being healthy is attractive. But the benefits of being healthy far exceed attractiveness and weight. If you are eye-locked on the scale and on your stomach in the mirror, you may feel discouraged early on when results aren't there yet. *It takes time for your body to show change.* If you put in the work consistently, results will follow. We're going to go about this in in a smart, mini-habit way to keep you on track regardless of your motivation, but remember this if you're having doubts.

3. High-intensity training requires recovery time. Be careful not to overdo high-intensity training, because an injury will set you back; more is not necessarily better.

4. You're not supposed to do high-intensity training every day (unless you're already an elite athlete). You know now from the studies that it doesn't require a lot of time exercising to make a difference. And here's the good news, depending on how you look at it: the more overweight you are, the more results you'll see from exercising.

5. High-intensity exercise keeps your body working, even after you stop. If the results of HIIT were limited to time spent exercising, it would be shown to be inferior to moderate-intensity exercise in studies. Instead, it's shown to be far superior, and that's because of the effect it has after you stop.

One workout I've been doing in my apartment building is interval training in the stairwell. (Very few people use the stairs in my building. Everyone takes the elevator. I digress.) Starting at the bottom, I sprint up the stairs as fast as I can. Then I'll "actively rest" by going back down the stairs at a pace that lets me catch my breath. Pro tip: I play the Rocky Balboa theme song on my phone, and put it at the top of the stairs, so as the difficulty increases toward the top and I'm feeling fatigued, the music gets louder to cheer me on!

One day after I had finished interval training session on the stairs, I continued to *actively sweat* for 10 minutes. Even after I took a shower, I continued to sweat. My body was still working. A study found this "afterburner" effect for fat oxidation: "Although more lipid was used during exercise in the low-intensity trial, more lipid was used after the high-intensity exercise."[162]

To conclude, when you exercise for fat loss, don't aim for time, aim for intensity. You can easily make up your own HIIT program. The basic idea is to go all out in an exercise for 15-60 seconds with a period of rest of 1-5 minutes.

If you want to use the treadmill, most of them have an interval setting. When I use the treadmill or exercise bike, I tend to adjust the speed manually. One good idea for an entertaining interval session is to watch a TV show or game (if your gym has a TV) and, whenever a commercial comes on, go all-out for its duration. Commercials take up roughly five to seven minutes total out of a 30-minute show, which is a nice interval split. When your show comes back on, you'll be rewarded with rest and entertainment at once! It's a nice little system that I've enjoyed. My friend and I have also done "curl challenges" during commercials, in which we curl a relatively light weight for the full duration of the commercial break.

The internet has plenty of other ideas for high-intensity training. Search for "HIIT workouts" or "interval training," and make it fun! You'll see interval training as a mini habit option in the next section.

Walking

Walking is *very* good. If you look at the human body, it's easy to see that we're meant to walk. In the past, walking was necessary to get around. We've since invented our way out of having to walk very much, but walking is too good for us to quit doing.

If you want to start out with something effective and not intimidating, walking is a proven winner. Whereas most exercise is known to increase appetite, one study found that the energy deficit induced by walking did not result in increased appetite: "This study demonstrates that, despite inducing a moderate energy deficit, an acute bout of subjectively paced brisk walking does not elicit compensatory responses in acylated ghrelin, appetite, or energy intake. This finding lends support for a role of brisk walking in weight management."[163]

The National Weight Control Registry says that, among people who have achieved lasting weight loss, walking is the most commonly reported form of exercise.[164] Anecdotally, I've found that lots of walking makes my stomach trimmer, more so than resistance exercise. I highly recommend making walking your "base" activity, and then doing HIIT as a bonus. You can combine them into one by aiming to walk a certain amount and then doing the occasional run/sprint. I'm aware of how unstructured that sounds, but structured routines are for people who already have strong exercise habits.

If you are still in the stages of fighting yourself to exercise, a structured "full workout" plan will be a great struggle to do consistently. Consider unstructured plans like "walk to the end of the driveway, optionally continue walking, and optionally do interval sprints during the walk." The difficulty is adaptable to you, meaning that you have very little reason to say no to it, even on your "off" days.

Resistance Training

Resistance training is the best way to increase lean muscle mass. This is highly beneficial for a number of reasons, but it has not been studied very much in regards to weight loss. Theories abound about how more muscle mass increases metabolism, but one study found that aerobic training was superior for weight loss, because resistance training did not result in fat loss (it did result in lean muscle mass gains).[165] Starting out, I recommend focusing on walking and aerobic (HIIT) exercise. Those are going to give you the greatest initial return on time and energy invested.

That said, resistance training is more useful than aerobic exercise for daily living. It can improve your posture and your performance in anything active, and it can even reduce pain caused by weakness or help you recover from injury (physical therapy). Don't rule it out completely! It's fun to see yourself get stronger with weight progression. If you learn to enjoy exercise, you'll love resistance training.

Fitness Mini Habits

If you've never been able to exercise consistently, you've got to try having an exercise mini habit. These are just some of the fitness mini habits you could create. There are certainly more! Most of these mini habits take *seconds*, not minutes or hours. The busiest person on Earth has time for this. The laziest person on Earth has enough energy for this. Mini habits make exercise unintimidating, fun, and always doable (the opposite of nearly every exercise program). Here's the list of fitness mini habits.

- One push-up
- One pull-up
- One sit-up
- 10 jumping jacks
- Run in place for 30 seconds
- Run on a treadmill for 30 seconds
- Dance for one song
- Run up and down a flight of stairs one time
- Walk beyond the end of your driveway or mailbox
- Put on your gym clothes (seriously)
- Put on your gym clothes and do one push-up (or other exercise)
- "Show up" at the gym without specific exercise plans (please try it before you discount it)
- One intense exercise interval lasting 30 seconds (sprinting, stairs, running in place as fast as you can, etc. Since you can do this running in place, you can do it anywhere!). Alternatively, you can do moderate-intensity exercise for 30 seconds.
- Press play on a workout video (or aim to complete 30 seconds of a workout video)
- Stand up to work once every two hours (if you have a stand-up desk), or get up for a few seconds every hour to wake up your metabolism if you only have a sitting desk.

Fitness Bonus: Do more of the same exercise or more of a different exercise.

You may notice some variations, like putting on gym clothes vs. putting on gym clothes AND doing an exercise mini habit vs. showing up at the gym. For some, doing an exercise when they aren't in workout clothes is futile for bonus reps, because they don't want to exercise in business clothes. That's why there's a "put on gym clothes" mini habit, which may be enough to start the exercise process. Others may need to begin exercising in order to get the process started, but also need to be in workout gear, so, for them, the ideal mini habit is going to be something like "put on gym clothes and do one push-up." Yet others will do well with just a "one pull-up" type of mini habit. I started with one push-up per day, and now I aim to "just show up" at the gym, which has worked really well.

Offbeat Mini Habit (not related to exercise or food)
Meditate for one minute: Meditation is one of the best indirect practices for weight loss, because it improves many relevant areas. It can decrease cortisol levels, improve your willpower, increase your mindfulness and focusing ability, and help you sleep better. Each of these has been shown to help with weight management. Meditating for just one minute can make a difference. Try it! Search for "one minute meditation" on YouTube for a guided meditation session.
Bonus: Meditate another minute or seven.

8

Mini Habit Plans

Everyone Laughs until They Experience the Results

"Do the difficult things while they are easy and do the great things while they are small. A journey of a thousand miles must begin with a single step."
~ Lao Tzu

Mini Habit Cues

Now we will bring it all together into a strategy that fits your lifestyle like a glove. Here's a recap of the mini habit ideas we've covered so far. Choose a maximum of four you'd like to integrate into your life.

Food Mini Habits
- Eat one (extra) serving of fruit
- Eat one (extra) serving of vegetables
- Make one mini healthy food upgrade
- Prepare one healthy meal at home
- Drink one glass of water
- Chew each bite 30+ times

Fitness Mini Habits
- One push-up
- One pull-up
- One sit-up
- 10 jumping jacks
- Run in place for one minute
- Run on a treadmill for one minute
- Dance for one song
- Run up and down a flight of stairs one time
- Walk beyond the end of your driveway or mailbox
- Put on your gym clothes (seriously)
- Put on your gym clothes and do one push-up (or other exercise)
- "Show up" at the gym without specific exercise plans (please try it before you discount it)
- One intense exercise interval lasting 30 seconds (sprinting, stairs, running in place as fast as you can, etc. Since you can do this running in place, you can do it anywhere!). Alternatively, you can do moderate intensity exercise for 30 seconds.
- Press play on a workout video (or aim to complete 30 seconds of a workout video)
- Stand up for a small amount of time while working (stand-up desk) or get up for a few seconds every hour to wake up your metabolism. I find with stand-up desks, it's often better not to aim for a set amount of time, but to "just stand up for a moment to work." Then I turn the music on, groovin' as I work.

Offbeat Mini Habit
Meditate for one minute

Visit minihabits.com for more mini habit ideas.

In the first *Mini Habits* book, I covered the basic strategy of using small daily practices to create mini-sized habits and change your behavior. Once you commit to a mini habit, it's important to define your cue.

Mini Habit Cues
A habit cue is whatever triggers you to perform the behavior. For example, a person wanting to develop a guitar practicing habit might say, "I will practice playing guitar every day at 7:30 PM." The cue is 7:30 PM.

I have good news. Weight loss is challenging, but when it comes to forming good eating habits, you have a significant advantage over other behaviors. Meals themselves are cues. For example, one push-up can be done at 6 PM (time cue), before a shower (activity cue), or any time during the day (flexible daily, no specific cue). A meal, however, is going to happen whenever it happens, and your mini habit will be in play whenever it does (i.e., a meal-based mini habit's cue is the meal itself).

Therefore, every meal-based mini habit will have an activity-based cue. The one exception is if you decide to use the flexible daily cue for all of your mini habits. In that case, you'd complete your mini habits at any time during the day, even between meals.

My mini habits have always been the flexible "do it any time before you go to sleep" type, because I am literally the least schedule-driven person I know. I rarely make plans. I'm not "busy." Almost every day is freestyle for me, and as long as I get the right things done, I'm happy. This lifestyle choice allows me to do things like travel at a moment's notice. To me, not having things on the schedule is freedom (one of humanity's longstanding core desires).

Here's why I bring that up: Most self-help advice ignores people like me, or else they suggest that I should transform myself into a "type A" person. I see the advantages of living that way, but there are also advantages to my way and other ways of living. Poor strategies force you to adapt to them (e.g., dieting); smart strategies adapt themselves to where you are right now. This book has a smart strategy flexible enough to fit the lifestyle of all types of people (A, B, C, R, and Alien).

There are three cues to choose from: activity-based, time-based, and the flexible "any time before bed" option. If you're schedule-driven, you'll do well with the time- or activity-based cues. If you live a spontaneous and non-scheduled lifestyle, you'll love the flexible daily cue. That said, there are no hard rules about who can succeed with what cue. Maybe schedule-driven people would enjoy the opportunity to find a time between activities to squeeze in a mini workout. Maybe spontaneous people would enjoy a bit more structure in their lives with scheduled mini habits. All of these cues can work, but make sure you choose one for each mini habit (except meals, which we'll cover next).

Activity-Based Cue: These actions are cued by activities you know you'll be doing each day. Example of four activity-based mini habits: Eat one serving of fruit once you arrive at work, eat one serving of vegetables during your first work break, drink one glass of water when you get home from work, and chew each bite 30 times during your daily work snack. (A clever activity cue for exercise is to do at least one push-up or alternative exercise action after you use the restroom. That is more than once per day, but that's still doable for some people.)

Time-Based Cue: Time-based actions can work well if you have a tightly scheduled lifestyle in which every moment is planned for. Example of three time-based mini habits: Eat one healthy snack at 3:15 PM, drink one glass of water at 6 PM, and eat a bowl of fruit at 7 PM.

Flexible Daily Option (No Cue): These actions can be done whenever, as long as you do them before the day ends. They're flexible, but they require a bit more mindfulness, as you have to choose when to do them each day rather than rely on a preset cue. Example of four flexible mini habits: Eat one serving of fruit any time before bed, eat one serving of vegetables before bed, chew each bite 30 times at any meal during the day, and drink one glass of water before bed.

Traditionally, only time-based and activity-based cues are possible for forming habits, but a mini habit is so small and easy to do that it doesn't need a specific cue. We don't need cues for bad habits, do we? We just tend to do them at various times because they're easy and rewarding. A mini habit has the same sort of appeal, only it's a good habit.

A smoker may smoke when eating, drinking, and/or stressed out. That's multiple cues for one behavior. In the same way, you'll develop some triggers for a flexible daily mini habit, but won't rely on any one cue. There are still triggers involved, but you'll let them grow "in the wild."

The advantage of this is diversified strength. Think of a cue as an individual root. You can develop one very strong root for a habit, or you can build a number of weaker roots. Multiple-root habits have individually weaker roots, but together, they may be more resilient than a one-root habit. This is precisely why bad habits are difficult to break—because it's not as if you can just single out the one trigger for the bad behavior and avoid it. The triggers are numerous, and some of them are even internally triggered by certain feelings (unavoidable).

With a mini habit, you can harness this power for good. It's why I write every day, but not at any specific time. It's why I exercise almost daily, but not on a schedule. To help you decide between these three cue options, here's a table that shows the strengths and weaknesses of each cue.

Benefits	Cues		
	Time "at 4 pm sharp"	**Activity** "after breakfast"	**Deadline** "anytime before bed"
Flexibility	1	2	5
Remembering	5	4	2
Time To Habit	5	5	1
"Never Lose"	2	3	4
Bonus Reps	3	3	3
Multiple Habits	3	4	5
Requires	discipline, reliable reminders	mindfulness of trigger activities	mindfulness, commitment to focus on building mini habits

Each cue is ranked from 1 to 5 in various categories, 5 being the best possible score. Here's what the categories mean.

Flexibility is how much freedom you have in deciding when to perform the behavior.

Remembering is how conducive the cue is to helping you remember to do the behavior. A time-based cue is inflexible because you must complete it at a specific time, but it helps you to remember because you can put it on your calendar or set a reminder on your phone. The flexible daily plan has no concrete, single cue, meaning it's the easiest one to forget. You can use reminders with any cue. For the flexible cue, try placing a pen on your pillow to remind you to do your mini habit before bed (or better yet, place a sticky note reminder in the fridge for your food-based mini habits).

Time to habit is the speed at which your behavior will form neural pathways and become habitual. Activity- and time-based cues will become habits faster, because they have only one pattern for the brain to recognize. If you choose a flexible daily plan, you might develop several go-to cues, and multiple behavioral patterns will take longer for the brain to solidify into habit. Flexible habits are structured a lot like "wild" habits that we form unintentionally. Smokers don't decide to smoke at 11 PM every day, they smoke after various triggers (multiple cues). Multiple cues make it difficult to break bad habits; in the same way, when your good habits have multiple cues, they have better "stickiness," as they aren't dependent on one cue.

"Never lose" is the ability to successfully complete your mini habits every day and well—never lose. It's most difficult with a time-based cue, because if you miss your cue at 2 PM, you technically failed. With a daily cue, you have all day to succeed, even if you do it right before bed. That's not to say that it is difficult to always win with a time-based cue, only that it's relatively more difficult than with a flexible cue.

Bonus reps is the likelihood that you'll do more than your mini requirement. Each cue is about equal in this regard.

Multiple habits is the ease with which each cue supports multiple habits. Any of the cues can do well with multiple habits, but the flexible plan is strongest here, since you can adapt your daily habits to the flow of your day.

The best plan is the one that works for and appeals to you. All of my mini habits use the flexible daily requirement, because it suits my unscheduled lifestyle. You might not know which style suits you best right away, so don't be afraid to experiment. You can mix and match cues as well. For example, maybe you set the goal to drink at least one glass of water per day (flexible daily), but also require one serving of vegetables at dinner (activity), and a raw carrot at 3:15 PM (time). In general, it's probably best to choose one type of cue across all of your mini habits for simplicity, but again, the only "rule" is to do what works best for you.

If you prefer, you can just use this system by choosing up to four mini habits (and a cue for each). Alternatively, you can choose a "meal plan" for all of your food-related mini habits.

Meal Plans

These meal plans all use activity-based cues (the meal itself) and have different objectives for those meals. The strategies below share the same life-changing concepts we've been discussing, but their implementation is flexible to suit you.

Make sure you only choose ONE of these plans. These are competing options, not a checklist. Think of these as themes to help you remember when and how to complete your food-based mini habits. If you go with one of these meal plans, don't forget to add on a fitness mini habit using one of the cues from the last chapter.

1. The Meal Upgrade Plan

This is my favorite strategy. In the meal upgrade plan, you choose one mini habit "upgrade" to do at every single meal you eat. This means that, even if you're eating an unhealthy fast food meal, it's not a total loss as you might typically see it. You can choose to chew each bite 30 times, drink water instead of soda, drink a glass of water before eating, get a lettuce wrap instead of the bun, or swap your fries for a healthier side. To determine what counts as a healthy upgrade, use your past behavior as a marker. If you already always drink water, that's fantastic, but don't count it as an upgrade.

The strength of this plan is that you won't need to keep track of what you've done. Every meal serves as your cue to perform one small healthy "upgrade" to the way you'd typically eat. Bonus (always optional): You can make additional upgrades at any meal, or go for a giant upgrade by eating a fully healthy meal.

With this choice, you'll form the habit of looking for small healthy upgrades when you eat, which is probably the most valuable habit to form for weight loss. You will be less likely, however, to form specific healthy habits like drinking water before meals, eating particular fruits or vegetables, and so on, because your healthy upgrade could vary with every meal.

For traveling, this is a good option, since it gives you complete flexibility and keeps you mindful of your eating habits.

2. The Meal Stronghold Plan

The goal here is to conquer one meal at a time. All of your efforts will be focused on one meal, and your other meals will be whatever you want. If you choose this plan, start with breakfast. All of your mini habits, such as adding or swapping fruits or vegetables for your usual meal, chewing your food 30 times or more, or drinking water before or during eating, will be done for this meal. Once you find yourself eating healthy food, chewing it well, and drinking water for breakfast consistently with a long winning streak, you can move on to lunch. I don't recommend you do so before at least two months have passed, because if you switch to lunch too soon (before your breakfast behavior is habitual), you risk trying to do too much too soon, which all former dieters know ends in failure.

This is called the stronghold plan, because one meal will become your stronghold for living a healthy lifestyle. If you can permanently transform the way you eat one meal, you can do the same for all meals. Though slightly different from the traditional mini habits setup, this is still progress every day, and it will be a great foundation to build from. Choosing breakfast first is a good idea, because how you start the day can greatly influence how you finish it. When you begin each day by eating well, it might just influence your lunch and dinner decisions, even though they are "eat whatever you want." Since there's no pressure to eat *every meal* perfectly, you will be able to maintain success at breakfast.

Mini Stronghold Example: Drink one glass of water between waking up and eating breakfast, eat one serving of fruit or vegetables at breakfast, chew each bite 30 times at breakfast, and do whatever you want for lunch and dinner. You might also consider creating healthy go-to meals, like full-fat yogurt and fruit for a quick breakfast (it's just as fast as cereal, only healthier) or eggs and spinach when you have time to cook.

3. The 2x2 Meal Plan

In this plan, you'll pick two meals per day to do the following: Eat one serving of healthy food (vegetables or fruit in most cases) and one meal modifier (drink a glass of water before meal, chew count, eat to 80% fullness, etc.). That's one healthy food and one modifier at two of your daily meals.

Two mini habits at two meals is four mini habits. When you add in your fitness mini habit, it makes five total mini habits, which is higher than I typically recommend. In this case, I think it's doable for *some* people, since two of these mini habits are modifications of behaviors rather than new behaviors (and so they should be even easier than most mini habits). If you struggle with this plan, it's probably because five mini habits is too many.

Choose Two Example: For breakfast, you drink a glass of water and eat a grapefruit. At dinner, you chew each bite 30 times and eat a side salad.

This is a flexible approach, because it doesn't specify the exact food or modifier to perform at each meal. You might use an approach like this while traveling, since traveling generally requires more flexibility.

4. The Line Drive Plan
This plan is simple and easy to remember. At every meal, perform the same mini habit of your choice. For example, you can drink a glass of water before every meal or during any meal as your main beverage choice. Drinking water instead of soda alone can have a big impact on your weight and health. Another option is to eat a side of vegetables at each meal, or even a specific vegetable if you have a favorite (but availability could make that a challenge). This plan isn't typically flexible, since you're picking a single specific action, but you can choose a backup action in case your primary choice isn't doable (such as a restaurant not serving your chosen vegetable).

Line Drive Example: Drink only water at every meal (assuming you eat three meals a day, this would count as three mini habits).

5. The Flexible Mini Plan
This plan means not having a meal plan. You will choose when to do your mini habits, whether it's eating a serving of fruit or making one healthy upgrade. In the flexible plan, you can freely choose to do your mini habits all in one meal, do two for breakfast and one for lunch another day, or any other combination. You could even accomplish them in between meals. Meals are the bulk of the food we eat, so I would still attempt to prioritize meals if you go this route.

Let's say you have three meal mini habits: one healthy upgrade, eat a serving of fruit, and chew each bite 30 times. On Sunday, you eat yogurt with blueberries, bananas, and strawberries instead of your regular cereal and milk. The yogurt is a "mini upgrade" over milk (probiotics and gut health), and your multiple servings of fruit meet your daily fruit goal and then some. That's two of three. You eat fast food for lunch. For dinner, you have steak and potatoes, and chew each bite 30 times (and a few more chews for the steak). That's three for three. Success!

The Final Word on Meal Plans
Choose only **one** of these meal plans to do at a time. You can choose an alternate meal plan for traveling, but otherwise, pick one plan and be consistent with it. This is what will change your brain and help you develop better habits that can benefit you for a lifetime.

Your chosen strategy here will serve as your core food strategy, but there's also fitness, snacking, meditation, and other non-meal mini habits to consider. Don't forget about them! I recommend adding a fitness mini habit to your meal plan, with an activity-based, time-based, or flexible daily cue. For simplicity's sake and for "healthy living synergy," you might consider using meals as the cue for your exercise mini habit as well (e.g., one push-up before dinner). I would suggest doing it before your meal, since exercising immediately after eating is rarely a fun experience.

If you think these plans aren't "enough," you're probably still thinking in terms of dieting, and you're discounting the power of real, long-term change. Consider this: Once you develop a healthy eating habit, *it becomes effortless*, and you can build from it. Most people underestimate the power of this because it isn't flashy; it just works. Dieting fails because it's too much at once for the brain and the body. This is the right dose of change that can sneakily make you stronger.

Now that we've discussed the general structure of how you'll be integrating positive changes into your life, let's discuss some of the questions you may still have.

Tracking

Tracking your progress is important for three reasons: it proves your commitment, encourages you daily, and lets you know exactly how well you're doing over time.

Here are some strategies for tracking your progress. In whatever strategy you choose, I recommend that you check off your success before you go to sleep. If you check off your task early in the day, the sense of completion might make you feel less motivated to do "bonus reps." Also, it's a good habit to check it off before bed so that you don't forget.

The Big Calendar (Recommended)
This is the strategy I use for tracking my mini habits. I use a large desk calendar on the wall in my room. I write my mini habits on a nearby dry erase board, and check off every day on the calendar when I complete them. It's simple and it works great. Checking off a successful day still feels great after months of mini habits!

Another option is a yearly "at a glance" calendar if you're just going to be checking off days. And a smart budget move is to print one of the many free printable calendars you'll find online (tip: simply print out your Gmail calendar). Physically making a check mark makes your success feel more tangible than digital tracking does. Additionally, if you put it in a prominent place where you'll see it often, it's going to make you mindful of your mini habits, your progress, and your success. Don't underestimate the impact of this!

The only excuse for breaking the chain of successful days is forgetting, because mini habits are too easy to fail. But forgetting is a poor excuse too, because your calendar will be in plain sight and every night before bed you'll ask, "Did I do my mini habits today?" And just to throw this out there, your mini habits don't have to be a fad you'll drop in a few months, this can be a *lifetime* pursuit. It works too well and is too flexible to quit!

Both writing down your mini habits initially and checking them off as you go is **vital** to your success. Don't skip it. Regardless of how you *track* your mini habits completion, I suggest you at least handwrite the habits themselves in a place you can see.

App Tracking
Some people will want to use their smartphone, and while I prefer the old-fashioned way, smartphones have some significant advantages. The first is accessibility—people carry their smartphones with them everywhere, even on vacations overseas. The second advantage is in visibility and reminders—some apps can remind you to do your mini habits, or serve as a concrete cue to take action.

Visit http://minihabits.com/tools/ for the updated list of recommended apps.

Final Note About All Digital Apps
You're going to see ideas for pre-made healthy habits to add from these apps and websites. Resist the urge to start these habits unless they are already minified (unlikely). If you really like one of them, make sure that you minify it before adding it to your repertoire! It looks fun to try doing 100 push-ups per day, but it's less fun when you quit. It's more fun to have one push-up per day as a goal and blow that tiny goal away for 200+ days in a row.

Rolling for Mini Habits

The following technique can be integrated into your mini habit plan however you wish (or not at all). You can even use this fun method to choose all of your mini habits each day. It's up to you. If you have trouble choosing between several options, you'll love this!

On a piece of paper or on your phone, list and number six of the same type of mini habit (food or fitness). For example, you might write this list for a fitness mini habit:

1. One push-up
2. One sit-up
3. 10 jumping jacks
4. Run in place for 30 seconds
5. Walk to the end of your driveway
6. Dance for one song

Make sure the list is somewhere that you'll see it daily—your desk, the refrigerator, an app in your phone, and so on. When you're ready to do a mini habit, get one die or two dice (or a dice rolling app).

With One Die
If you're using one die, roll it every day, and do the mini habit that corresponds to the number you roll. If your list was the one above and you rolled a five today, you would then walk to the end of your driveway. This gives you two opportunities for bonus reps: you can walk further than your driveway, or you can roll again!

IMPORTANT: one list takes the place of only ONE of your mini habits. You'll still only do one of these per day. If you really like this idea, you can create up to four lists (for four mini habits) to roll for each list to determine what you do that day.

With Two Dice

If you're using two dice, you have the option of expanding your list to 12 activities and doing what number you roll. Alternatively, you can keep the list at six mini habits and give yourself an either/or choice. If you roll a three and a four for this list, you'd choose between 10 jumping jacks and running in place for 30 seconds. If you roll a double six, then you must dance!

Optional Features

You can consider adding one difficult action to the list. For example, maybe you would put "run one mile" as number one, so if you roll a one, you'd have to run a mile. That isn't a mini habit, but it does add some stakes to the roll, and it makes your other mini habits seem *really* easy by comparison (a good thing!).

If you add a difficult challenge, you might consider adding some kind of reward to another number. For example, you could make six a "free choice," roll in which you choose your mini habit. Or you could keep six at "dance to one song" and add a small piece of candy as a bonus for rolling six. (See minihabits.com for more reward ideas.)

Rolling Benefits

The randomness of the dice rolls is fun and varies your activities, both of which can keep your experience fresh and enjoyable. While your daily behaviors will be more varied with this method (which seems like a hindrance for habit formation), you'll still form the habit of making progress in fitness and eating every day. Your primary goal is to change your relationship with the concepts of being active and eating healthy food, and this can accomplish that.

By rolling the dice to determine your next move, you actually decrease resistance to action even more. Rolling the dice is a contract in which you agree to do what it says. This is a diluted version of making a bet with a friend: "If they lose, I'll go in the dunk tank, but if they win, you have to buy me dinner." Someone might not volunteer for the dunk tank (where someone throws a ball at a target and you fall in the water if they hit it), but if it's a part of a friendly bet, they'll do it. The dice roll is a fun bet you make with yourself. Whatever it rolls, you do.

Lastly, the dice roll makes it easier to make a decision. Instead of deciding to do something you might find slightly uncomfortable (a fitness mini habit), you only have to decide to roll the dice, which starts the process of your mini habit.

Incorporating dice into your mini habits plan adds one more step, which is typically a bad thing, but the benefits and fun it provides are well worth it. For those who've seen weight loss as a lot of work and misery, this sort of "gamification" might be just what they need to succeed.

Mini Habits Troubleshooting

If you have problems making mini habits work for you, look no further.

I'm feeling resistance.
Resistance is a sign that your subconscious is uncomfortable with what you want to do. Run through this checklist to make sure your perspective is correct.

Am I aiming for a mini habit, or am I pretending to aim for a mini habit while secretly aiming for more? You cannot fool your subconscious mind, so don't try. Your *intention* needs to be small. Remember, it's one step at a time. This is not to say that you won't ever do more; it's to say that you'll get there most often by thinking in small, incremental steps, not by saying "I'll take this small step" and secretly requiring more of yourself.

Is my mini habit actually mini-sized? One of the biggest issues I've seen with mini habit implementation is that people don't minify the action enough. For example, someone will tell me they're struggling to read 10 pages in a book per day. Well, my mini habit is to read *two* pages per day, which is five times less! Ten pages might not sound like much, but on a bad, unmotivated day, it can be too much. Make your mini habits small, and you won't resist them. Consistency is much more important than quantity, which is why we make these mini-sized in the first place.

Do I still feel resistance? It's okay to feel some resistance, because you have willpower at your disposal. These mini behaviors are so small that there

172

should never be a time that you don't have enough willpower to force action. That's how this strategy is designed for success. Willpower is reliable, as long as you have enough of it for the action you want to take. Relying on how you feel is not a winning strategy. The most successful people in *any* field did not get there by only taking action when they felt like it. They show up every day, regardless of how hard life is. With a typical goal, this falls into the "easier said than done" category. With mini habits, this is easily said AND done. It doesn't matter what you've been through—you can drink a glass of water, eat an apple, or do a push-up!

Whenever you feel resistance toward a mini habit, be sure to challenge yourself on it. Don't accept that you don't feel like dancing for a minute. Think about how easy it would be and how you'd feel good about accomplishing it. Challenge yourself to get up and try it. The more you practice overcoming that initial resistance into an easy mini habit, the more you'll trust the process, and the better your results will be.

I've been skipping my mini habits.
Ask yourself these questions.

Am I taking this seriously? Look, I know that "chew your food 30 times" sounds goofy when you want to lose 100 pounds. But there's some irony here. The crash diets and boot camps seem like a serious effort to change your life, but they're actually aiming much lower than we are. They're a joke compared to the permanent life change possible with mini habits. A crash diet or boot camp aims for a short-term and superficial change in body composition. We're aiming deeper. We're aiming to *change your brain* and the way you relate to and think about food and exercise. People temporarily adhere to these insane, torturous programs because they are desperate for the promised results. If you can understand how much greater the result of lasting habitual change will be, you won't have any problem taking your daily mini habits seriously. This doesn't mean you won't laugh at "having to walk to the end of my driveway;" it only means that you'll be sure to do it, regardless of how silly it seems on the surface.

Do I have the right cues? If you're not getting it done for any reason, take a hard look at the cues you've chosen. If you chose a time- or activity-based cue, then maybe you need more flexibility and should try a flexible daily cue. If you have a flexible daily cue and keep putting it off or forgetting, then maybe you need a more structured cue (time or activity).

Do I have too many mini habits? Regardless of what I say, I know some people will immediately begin 10 mini habits after reading this book (I recommend four maximum). One guy told me he had some trouble completing his 20+ mini habits every day.

When you have too many mini habits, you overwhelm yourself by the *number* of things you must do, and the result is the same as for any overwhelming goal (failure). That being said, if you have four mini habits, that might *still* be too many for you. Personally, I do best with two or three mini habits. When I add in the fourth one, it doesn't work very well. And I'll add that I started with just *one* mini habit (one push-up per day) that completely transformed my life and relationship with exercise. So don't think that having only one mini habit is useless! If you aren't completing your mini habits, consider dropping one of them.

What if I complete some mini habits and not others?
Partial completion is failure in mini habits. These behaviors are supposed to be so easy that you can complete them all on the worst day of your life. So if you find yourself completing some, but not others, either drop the others or figure out why they're posing such a challenge to you. With all of the strategic plans for implementation, you can also try tweaking your mini habit plan to see if that helps. This strategy is meant for 100% daily success, but you might not achieve that immediately, as you figure out the strategy and number of mini habits that work for you. The great upside to having mini habits is the ease of restarting a mini habit program at any time for any reason. If you "fall off the horse," you can get back on within five minutes! Aim for 100% completion of all of your mini habits. If you're not hitting that mark, make adjustments until you do.

I never do bonus reps. What am I doing wrong?
Bonus reps are just that—a bonus. If you never go "above and beyond," there's no need to panic. Some habits take longer to take root than others. For example, my reading mini habit was fairly slow developing, my push-up mini habit had moderate growth, and my writing mini habit took off like a racehorse. You can expect variance, but otherwise, consider this.

Is your mini habit too small? This is something I didn't mention in the first *Mini Habits* book because I wasn't aware it was possible. One day, I received an email from a reader. She told me that she had written only 30 words in 30 days—one word per day. This gave me an epiphany: A mini habit is too small if the action fails to start the process of your target behavior.

For example, if your goal is to write more, writing just one word does not begin the writing process, because, at the very least, writing requires you to form a thought or phrase that means something. Otherwise, you can write "The" and stop thinking about it. My writing mini habit is 50 words per day, because that almost always leads to more ideas and writing; it begins the writing process. Since it's only a paragraph, I'm never intimidated by it. I don't get writer's block.

One push-up per day is a good example of a very small mini habit that's still enough to start the process of exercise. Once you get into push-up position and do one, it's conducive to doing more. Some people may feel the need to be in workout clothes before they exercise, so they might modify their habit to "change into gym clothes" or "change into gym clothes *and* do one push-up" or "change and drive to the gym."

One day, I noticed that every time I set up my doorway pull-up bar, I did pull-ups. From that moment on, I didn't set the goal to do even one pull-up; my goal was to set up the bar. Then habit took over.

Whatever the mini habit, pay close attention to what starts the process for you. If your mini habit is to eat a baby carrot and you only ever eat one, try making it two baby carrots to see if that gets the carrot party started. The ideal mini habit is always going to be at the level of lowest possible resistance that also begins the process of the target behavior.

Questions and Answers

What if I miss a day?
If you miss a mini habit for whatever reason, it's not a big deal. At all. A study on habit formation found that one day missed did not affect successful habit formation.[166] The only threat of missing a day is that you'll let it grow to two days (which is a new trend in the wrong direction). If you miss a single day, don't worry about it, but make it your highest priority to knock out your mini habits (early, if possible) the next day.

One advantage of having mini habits is the ease of "jumping back in" if you experience a setback. Since you can "get back on the wagon" in less than five minutes, you stand to succeed as long as you're committed to it.

Should I reward myself?

If you're familiar with the habit formation process (cue, behavior, reward), you might be expecting me to discuss rewards, but rewards are optional for mini habits. There is an intrinsic reward for accomplishing your goals, and that is plenty for a mini habit. Maybe we would need rewards to encourage a more difficult behavior, but a mini habit is easy enough to force yourself to do even without any external reinforcing reward. The intrinsic reward of success is enough for a mini habit. The only point in an external reward is to get your brain to the point that you're conditioned to do the behavior even without a reward, that is, you don't need a reward to do the behavior (which is one of the reasons it's superior!). As Sun Tzu said, "Victorious warriors win first and then go to war."

There's also a good reason not to think about rewards: It adds one more thing to manage. This strategy thrives on simplicity, so I recommend keeping it as simple as possible. That said, you can reward yourself and treat yourself well in general, and draw the connection to your success with mini habits. That's certainly worthwhile, but you don't need to make it a hard rule.

How many mini habits?

I recommend a maximum of four mini habits at a time. Aside from those, you'll have numerous (optional) opportunities to improve your health and weight. Don't worry about not doing enough! Besides building a foundation for lasting change, which already boosts this strategy above the rest, you're going to have opportunities to make short-term progress, too.

I remembered to chew each bite 30 times, but it was halfway through my meal. Does it still count?

Yes, it does. Chewing half of your meal 30 times per bite is a mini habit (you could even make it your standard mini habit if desired). The spirit of this strategy is that all progress is valuable. It's obviously better to remember to chew all bites 30 times, but if you're trying, give yourself the benefit of the doubt. The second most important thing (behind consistency) is to remain positive about your progress.

What is a healthy meal?

Healthy meals have one thing in common—they use real and minimally processed ingredients. They lack preservatives, added colors, added sweeteners, emulsifiers, added flavors, and other chemical additives. Beware of companies using these phrases to get your attention. Just because there are no artificial colors or flavors does not mean there aren't a lot of other terrible, processed ingredients. Healthy food is rare.

What counts as a serving of fruit?

When it comes to your mini habits, do not count any fruit that comes in a can or in sauce. Fresh or frozen fruit is easy to acquire almost anywhere, and it has plenty of flavor and sweetness on its own (it doesn't need the sugary syrup they put in fruit cups). If it's some kind of fruit salad with creamy dressing, whether you count that is up to you. My suggestion is not to cheat yourself either way. Your goal isn't to "cheat the system" and count a fruit snack pouch as your daily fruit; it's to eat more fruit! If you eat four blueberries covered in syrup or blueberry jam, that's not really hitting the mark.

What counts as a serving of vegetables?

The ideal target to hit here is raw vegetables. Second best is boiled, steamed, or baked vegetables. That said, if the only vegetables you'll eat are sauced beyond recognition or salted, you can start there. It's better to eat healthy food covered in unhealthy food than to only eat unhealthy food. So, if you only enjoy broccoli if it's smothered in something unhealthy, well, go for it.

The paltry, low-quality lettuce and tomato you might get on a fast food burger is better than nothing, but not what we're looking for. I suggest making the rule that vegetables need to "carry the most weight" in the food you're eating for it to count as a serving. French fries, for example, are potatoes, but that's dwarfed by the fact they're deep fried in vegetable oil.

If you want your vegetables to have more flavor, black pepper gives a healthy and delicious kick to basically any savory dish. There are many more spices that can do the same. I use organic all-purpose seasoning for most things. Healthy food is usually delicious as it is, but for some foods and some palates, experimentation might be warranted.

What if I don't like [insert healthy food here]?

You don't have to eat it if you don't like it. With the variety of flavors, textures, and preparations of fruits and vegetables, it's almost impossible to dislike everything. Find the combinations that work for you. I enjoy salads, blueberries, mangoes, strawberries, broccoli, and spinach the most, so I eat them the most. These foods are a small fraction of the number of options. I will occasionally eat cauliflower, but I don't care for it. I never eat mushrooms. Chicken is healthier than red meat, but I tend to go for beef and broccoli more often because I like how they go together. Remember that everything is on a scale, and that broccoli dipped in soybean oil ranch dressing is still healthier than macaroni and cheese.

What if I can't stop eating unhealthy food?
The strategy for temptations is in the next chapter. The sneak preview answer is: Don't try to willpower your way out of a poor diet. The way out of an unhealthy diet is not restriction, it's abundance! Unhealthy food provides a reward, and you must find an alternate way to get that reward. If you cut out a powerful reward completely, you won't last long!

You're going to continue to eat some unhealthy food as you integrate changes, and that's okay. The short-term perspective says that no amount of junk food is acceptable, and that just makes me want to eat a cheeseburger. Think abundantly, and move toward healthy food rather than away from unhealthy food. Our strategy in the next chapter is more specific and actionable than this advice, but perspective does matter.

What if I'm not in the mood for a carrot?
Just now, I took a break from writing to eat something. I thought about eating a carrot, but I was in the mood for something more substantial (like a meal). My desire for a full meal or heavy snack had discouraged me from eating "just a carrot." I suspect this feeling is *extremely* common, since vegetables are not calorie dense. In this case, I would usually skip the carrot and eat what I craved, but this time, I imagined actually eating the carrot. I thought about the flavor, texture, and satisfying crunch of it, and immediately, it became more appealing to me. But the key thought that sealed the deal was reminding myself that eating a carrot does not mean I can't eat something else too. I ate the carrot and enjoyed it. Not long after that, I once again desired a meal, but now I had a carrot in my stomach.

If you're in such a situation, you might think that eating the carrot was a "waste," since you still feel just about as hungry after eating it. This is NOT true. Vegetables provide powerful health benefits, independent of how well they sate your appetite. In addition, it's unlikely that your sense of hunger is so sensitive and accurate as to be able to say, "I feel exactly as hungry after eating the carrot as I did before." Did you measure your hunger before and after? What were the readings?

Vegetable consumption does not always have to be a "meal replacement." You can and should continue to eat if you're hungry. If you eat vegetables and you're still hungry, eat something else, even something unhealthy if you must. Abandon the dieting scarcity mindset. If you eat three whole carrots and a salad, and then eat a hot dog, dieting law says that you've failed. In reality, that is a huge success! If you hadn't eaten carrots and the salad, you might have eaten two or three hot dogs. But even if vegetables miraculously defied the laws of physics and didn't satisfy your appetite even a little bit, despite taking up space in your stomach and providing energy, they'd still be worth consuming for their many other health and weight loss benefits.

This is a vital perspective: Healthy foods might not be a 1:1 replacement for unhealthy foods in the early stages of your change. Eating a small salad might only satisfy 35% of your appetite, and of course you'll feel deprived if you think, "Darn. That salad was my meal but I'm still hungry. That pizza would have filled me up. I guess I must suffer to live healthy." No, no, no! That's so wrong that I hated typing it. You know what's better than three greasy slices of pizza? Three greasy slices of pizza plus a salad. If you're worried about the extra calories from the *salad*, well, just think about that.

When you eat something healthy, try not to have expectations for how it will affect your appetite. Don't make a light salad have to live up to the caloric satisfaction of a cheese steak sub. I call my salads "mega" for a reason! If you eat something healthy and you're still hungry, you can eat more of it or eat something else. That's all. Leave appetite regulation up to your body. Eat when hungry and stop when you're satisfied.

Is cheese fattening?
I don't believe that. Real cheese is a healthy food packed with nutrients. When you eat nacho cheese at a movie theater, that's not actually cheese. It might have cheese in it, but it has a lot more in it as well. When it comes to homemade nachos, the chips are far more fattening than the cheese (if it's real).

Cheese is basically in the same camp as milk, which we've discussed. It's not going to win "weight loss food of the year" awards, but it's not quite as bad as it's perceived to be either. As with milk, full fat cheese is the right choice. All of the science says that skim milk is more fattening and unhealthier than whole milk.

If foods like avocados (82% fat) and blueberries (high sugar) are not only helpful for weight loss, but two of the world's best weight loss foods, and studies suggest they are, it shows we need to stop caring so much about macronutrients and more about the quality of the entire food. The consistent finding in research is that processed foods make us fat—not high-fat foods, not high-sugar foods, processed foods.

In most cases, ultra-processed foods are stripped of life, low in fiber, low in satiety, low in bioavailable micronutrients, inflammatory, and high in calories, fat, and sugar. You can pinpoint any one of these areas and say, "That's it! We get fat because of low fiber foods!" But all of those roads lead us to the door of Frankenfoods. Foods designed in a lab are experiments, and, like any experiment, they can go poorly. While we don't get immediately sick from eating these foods, they confuse our bodies, starve us of nutrition, and make us fatter and disease-prone. Experiment failed. Let's go back to eating real food for our primary sustenance.

Should I buy organic?
It depends. I think it's funny how people take pro-organic and anti-organic stances on this issue, because whether or not to buy organic should be done on a case-by-case basis. I never buy avocados organic but I always buy berries organic. Why do you think that is?

The Environmental Working Group (in Washington, DC) tests produce for pesticide residue (pesticides are not used on organic produce). The top 15 most pesticide-laden foods for 2016 were (in order of most pesticides to least): strawberries, apples, nectarines, peaches, celery, grapes, cherries, spinach, tomatoes, sweet bell peppers, cherry tomatoes, cucumbers, snap peas, blueberries, and potatoes. These are the foods to buy organic to limit your pesticide consumption. The 10 foods least important to buy organic (because they tested for the least amounts of pesticides) are: avocado, sweet corn, pineapple, cabbage, sweet peas, onions, asparagus, mangoes, papaya, kiwi, and eggplant. The full list is on their website.[167]

Now, organic produce might contain more nutrition because of the way it's grown. For example, a study on milk found that "organic milk contained 25% less ω-6 fatty acids and 62% more ω-3 fatty acids than conventional milk."[168] That is a vastly superior ratio of fatty acids. But given the cost of organic and varying budgets, it's important to know where to begin. Produce is the most important *area* to buy organic, but not necessarily all produce. If your food budget is tight and you're buying organic avocados, well, you shouldn't!

What about GMOs? Genetic modification is another way humans have tampered with food. I'm not going to get into it much, but I try to avoid them when possible, which is most easily done by buying organic food. GMOs are a hotly debated issue, but when you're eating fast food every day, GMOs are the least of your concerns (actually, maybe they are a concern, since fast food is loaded with them). If you make healthy dietary changes, you'll automatically eat fewer GMOs, which is to say that GMOs are not the right focal point unless your diet is already healthier than 95% of the population.

Bonus Challenges

In this book, I'm introducing a new concept I call "mini challenges." They are like a mini habit in size, but they are optional and situational. These mini challenges are never required, and are not a part of your core mini habit plan. They are opportunities to make bonus progress.

Most dieting and weight loss programs are blinded by the thought of what would happen if adherence were perfect; they overload participants with rules and restrictions. But for a strategy to succeed, its mandatory requirements (i.e. rules) must be handled with great care to preserve autonomy and prevent burnout. Optional activities, however, can be practically unlimited without a negative impact, because any instance of *not* doing them will not harm your self-confidence or winning streak.

Do you see how exciting this is? Imagine a typical day. Rather than feeling overwhelmed by the gap between who you are and who you want to become, you'll have an *easy* list of daily mini habits to do, and additionally, you'll have a bigger list of small but impactful behavioral challenges to do if and when you desire. These aren't obligations, they are opportunities. Obligations are a burden, but opportunities are weightless and enticing.

These optional challenges (and your mini habits) will let you experience healthy living in a safe environment. Anyone who has dieted has experienced healthy living in a controlling, suffer-for-results environment.

This is, unfortunately, the most common perspective of "healthy living." It's weighed down by shame, reminders of past failures to adhere to diets, and other emotional baggage. Healthy living has never been the "fun uncle," but it can be fun if you experience it *on your terms* without its undeserved associations. Remove all of your preconceived notions, start experimenting, and you'll be surprised at how enjoyable this journey can be.

The common idea behind these mini challenges is this: Being active is worthwhile in any dose.

TV Challenge: Before watching TV, exercise or move for 20 seconds (jumping jacks, push-ups, jogging in place, dancing like a jester, etc.). Need a reminder? Attach one to your TV or remote. You can use a small mark or sticker, since you'll know what it stands for. If you think 20 seconds isn't worthwhile, I challenge you to test that theory right now. Get groovin' full speed for 20 seconds and see how you feel.

While 20 seconds is short, it will seem longer while you're in motion! Afterwards, your pounding heart will tell you exactly how "worthless" that 20 seconds was. I think 20 seconds is a good amount of time for this mini challenge, because the end is already in sight before you begin, and yet it's not over immediately once you start, which creates a nice mix of low resistance to action and a satisfying payoff. Low resistance and a satisfying payoff are a powerful formula for any behavior to stick (this formula is how bad habits thrive).

TV Challenge Bonus: For every 30 minutes of TV, get up and move for another 20 seconds. I recommend dancing to scare your family members. If you are watching TV with your family, and you randomly get up and start dancing without telling them why you're doing it, you are my friend for life.

TV Commercial Challenge: Every commercial you watch during TV, get up and move around. You don't even need to "exercise" per se, just get up and move around. Commercials are terrible anyway. Walk laps around the interior of your house. Clean part of your house. This will keep your metabolism from plummeting during a TV session, and it's a nice way to be entertained while doing something positive for your body! When your show comes back on, you'll feel great for "earning" more leisure time. It's small and sounds silly, but please try it before you discount it. It feels great.

It's not good to "earn" unhealthy food with healthy living, but it is VERY good to "earn" relaxation and entertainment for healthy living. Relaxation and entertainment aren't harmful; they are an *essential* part of healthy living and the natural reward for hard work. People often feel ashamed for watching too much TV, but that's because they do it inactively and in big chunks. If you add activity to your leisure time, you win on multiple levels because of the synergies. You'll enjoy your entertainment more because you won't be distracted by feeling "lazy shame."

Stairs Challenge: Whenever possible, take the stairs! Take pride in skipping the elevator and escalator. I am the only person in my apartment complex who lives on the 7th floor and takes the stairs. For different results, you must live and think differently than others. This is one opportunity to do so.

Be careful not to think in all-or-nothing terms. If your destination is the 18th floor, you can take three flights of stairs and then take the elevator. Or take the elevator and jog in place as you ascend (especially do this if there are others in the elevator with you). If there are several flights of escalators and stairs, take the stairs first and the escalator next. There are no rules. Nobody is going to say, "Hey! She just took the stairs and then switched to the escalator! How inconsistent! That's weird!"

Parking Spot Challenge: Park in the furthest spot from the store. The walk isn't that much farther, and you won't be hunting for "the best spot" for five minutes too long like everyone else. Here's a secret: The best parking spot is the farthest from the store, because it gives you the best walk, the most enjoyment of the weather, the least stress, and the most rewarding feeling.

Walking/Biking Challenge: If you can walk/bike somewhere instead of drive, go for it. I am often surprised at how enjoyable it can be to walk places.

9
Situational Strategies

Rules Can Be Broken. Strategies Are Forever.

"Everybody has a plan until they get punched in the mouth."
~ Mike Tyson

Strategies Overview

Dieters abide by their list of good and forbidden foods until life happens, and it turns out that it happens often. Such rules can be broken, but strategies last forever.

The following strategies are not rules to follow. These are in-the-moment mindsets and actions you can choose to use at any time. It's up to you if and when you'd like to use them. All of these strategies are conducive to influencing you and your decisions in the right direction. Since you don't *have* to use them, there's no feeling of "messing up" if you eat a popsicle on a whim.

The core mini habit plans we discussed in the previous chapter are the "main course." These are optional, but highly encouraged "side dishes." This reflects the nature of healthy living, which is mostly dictated by habit, and secondarily dictated by our perspective and the non-habitual choices we make every day.

Since real-world application is more important than theory, what follows is a list of several challenging real-world situations you'll find yourself in, with custom strategies to help you make winning choices more often.

Temptation Strategy: Mini Routines

You have a plan in place. It's fantastic. But then you're hit with a strong desire to sink your teeth into seven cookies … uh oh! What can you do? The worst thing you can do is resist the craving directly and deprive yourself.

A craving is a rare opportunity for progress. Do you know why? There's significant motivation behind your craving, and we can harness it! Motivation is the very thing billions of people want when it comes to their goals. Here we have it, and it's powerful, but it's motivation to eat a cookie, which isn't in line with our goals. How can we use this to our advantage?

I've used the tactic I'm about to tell you about to dramatic positive effect. One of my less impressive habits is bingeing on video games. I've played for double digit-hour sessions many times. (I told you I'm lazy.) Often, when I feel the urge to play, I will think about previous binges and tell myself *I shouldn't play* or *I shouldn't play too much* (does this sound like you with food?). These thoughts are shame-driven and make us feel deprived, which makes things worse.

I've found a better strategy than shame. Let's say that my overarching goal is to play games less and be more productive. To accomplish this when I'm tempted, I will place a small, non-intimidating, and beneficial obstacle between myself and my game. And I do it on the condition that I can play the game without shame. A no-shame game, if you will. On multiple occasions, this has led me to productive work sessions lasting several hours without playing any games. Other times, I've worked some and played some, coming out satisfied with each. Regardless of what happens when I do this, I win. Now, let's talk about what this strategy can do for you when unhealthy food temptation strikes. Aside from the core mini habit strategy, this may be the most exciting strategy in the book.

How to Be an Opportunistic Craver instead of a Victim
What's the typical behavior of a craver? They resist until they cave to the crave. They fight, exhaust themselves, lose, and eat the treat. It's as if they're *victims* of a craving attack. Then, they feel bad about losing the battle. What if these "victims" could not *merely* defend themselves from these craving attacks, but go on the attack themselves? We're going to completely change this game, and you will never look at your cravings in the same way again.

We'll start by asking you a piercing question. What's more harmful to your long-term weight loss goals: eating an unhealthy snack or *feeling ashamed* about eating an unhealthy snack? Which one do you think causes more weight gain over time? Put that thought on the back burner as we talk about cravings.

Think of your craving as a magnetic force, causing you to steadily move toward it. You can resist it for some time, but the moment you let your guard down, you'll rush in. Our strategy is to harness this force by putting some choice miniature obstacles *between* you and the craving. Not instead of the craving. Between you and the craving. But before we get into the mini obstacles, we must get our perspective right.

By completing these mini obstacles, you are indeed getting closer to your cookie (or whatever it may be). However, and this is extremely important, you are NOT "earning it." You are not doing these things in order to "buy" the right to eat something unhealthy. The concept of "buying" unhealthy food with healthy behaviors suggests that they cancel each other out, that they're worth the same, that a little bit of good makes up for a little bit of sin, and other similarly false beliefs. You are not buying the cookie, you're buying a "get out of shame free" card. If you complete your mini obstacles, you will agree to feel no shame about eating the item. (If you still feel shame, you ought to be ashamed of yourself! Actually, no, that wouldn't be good. You get the point. If you begin to feel shame, simply remind yourself of your deal.) If you complete this task, agree with yourself that you can eat your object of craving without shame.

If you're wondering why you would ever choose to complete these mini obstacles when you could just go for the treat directly, I like how you think. Question everything. This strategy is so good that you will gladly choose the package with mini obstacles on many occasions. And why? Because unlike the "straight to the cookie option," the mini obstacle package comes without any shame AND you still get your food. It's the same reason why I enjoy working before playing video games—whether or not I play after working, I feel good about my decision to do something positive and don't feel bad about playing video games.

Resisting food cravings directly is futile and harmful. Successful resistance today means that you're weaker tomorrow; resist the next day too, and you'll be even weaker the one after that. Direct resistance is the most common choice for dealing with temptation, but it is a proven loser for three reasons. First, it makes you feel deprived, and very few people can accept deprivation for long if given a choice. Second, it makes you focus on the temptation more: "I mustn't eat the chocolate" makes you think about the chocolate, increasing the strength of the temptation as you burn through your willpower. Third, it leads to shame if/when you cave, which is what we feel when we want to do "the right thing" but do the wrong thing instead. That last point is why you're not "earning" the treat, but earning a "shame free" outcome.

This is not a fight to resist your craving. It doesn't matter if you're able to resist your craving in any given moment, because the willpower war doesn't end there. If you win the cookie fight this morning, it may weaken you for the cheeseburger brawl at lunch, or the battle of cheesecake hill tonight. You may resist for an hour and then cave in. You may resist for *days or weeks*, and then binge on the 37th day. Temptation is a perpetually recurring threat, and this is why strategy is paramount and direct resistance is counterproductive. This strategy consistently increases your chance to beat the temptation without draining your willpower and making you feel deprived. You can replicate this strategy several times a day without issue, because even if you give in to the temptation, the act of going through this process strengthens you.

To summarize the correct perspective: Give yourself full permission to eat the item, without shame, without regret, and without any hint of self-judgment IF you go through the first two mini obstacles in the list I'm about to show you. This turns your motivation to eat the treat into a powerful motivator to do these mini challenges, because you're granting yourself immunity from shame with only a small, easy condition to meet. On the surface, it looks like you're giving yourself permission to gain weight and lose: *You're saying I do these easy little things and then I can eat this junk food without feeling bad about it? Are you crazy?!*

We are now face-to-face with the counterintuitive side of psychology, because as much as your shame-free pass to eat the cookie is appealing to the part of you that wants to eat alllll the cookies, dropping shame is *far more beneficial* to the "I want to eat healthy food to lose weight" part of you.

Let's put it all together now. The incentive (eating item without shame) that makes the motivator (eating item) even more desirable does you the great favor of decreasing your sense of shame (immediately) while motivating you to complete a highly beneficial mini routine that is designed to end with you *sometimes no longer wanting the item.* You may or may not end up consuming the item, but that's not the measure of victory. *The measure of victory is whether you've strengthened yourself or weakened yourself.* As for the question I asked earlier: Eating something unhealthy or even a binge session is a one-time event. The shame from eating one unhealthy item or one binge session can spiral and last *years.* Which one sounds like the bigger threat to you?

This mini routine itself is not merely going to make you more mindful, it's not merely going to strengthen your willpower and self-control; it's going to build you up instead of tear you down. It's not about the individual instance, it's about who you're becoming. You can "lose" to your craving and still make *significant* progress toward changing your behavior.

Do you see how powerful this is? Can you see the difference between this and "fat shaming," alternating starvation and bingeing cycles, and inflexible dieting? This is the refreshing difference that real strategy brings. It is superior to the smartest doctor in the world telling you exactly what foods to eat for weight loss.

Now, there's one more factor to consider. Whenever you are tempted and decide to take on this mini challenge, which I recommend you do as frequently as possible (since it's win-win), make your initial requirement to complete the first two actions. You'll notice that the list I give you is longer than two actions, and that's because you can choose to add additional challenges to your requirement. It's up to you! Just like the core mini habits strategy, it has a low floor and no ceiling.

What if you feel that your challenges weren't "good enough" to eat the item shame-free? First of all, congratulations, because you're finally fighting the correct enemy. The food isn't your problem, self-destructive behavior is, and shame is the heart of self-destructive behavior. I must remind you, however, that shame should *never* be involved with eating, since food isn't moral (good or bad); different foods just have varying effects on our bodies. Besides that, you can always do more of any challenge if you feel it's necessary, or you can move on to the next mini challenge. Whatever you decide, make it your goal to free yourself of shame.

Here are the challenges. I said they were obstacles before because they basically are obstacles in your path from A to B, but a more positive phrase for these is mini challenges.

Temptation Mini Routine
I've thought through the ordering, but you may respond better to a different ordering. I put meditation first to slow down the mind, increase mindfulness, delay the action, and calm emotions. This addresses several possible food triggers. It then progresses to substitution to satisfy biological cravings, exercise to activate your "live healthy" motivation, water to address thirst that is often confused for hunger, a small delay, another activity of your choice, a bribe, walking away, and finally, portion negotiation. Here they are in detail, using the example of a cookie craving.

1. Meditate for one minute. This is a good way to clear the mind and slow down. See it as delaying the cookie: *ok, I can eat the cookie, but first, I*

will meditate for a minute. This simple delay (and the impact of meditation) may be enough to make the craving disappear.

Sit down somewhere quiet. If you're at a party, excuse yourself to a quieter room, outside, or the restroom. Just focus on your breaths for a minute. Don't fight thoughts and desires, just observe them as if you're an outsider. Search for "one minute meditation" on YouTube for a guided session. Why is this #1? Meditating will reduce your stress immediately, improve your emotional state, and make you more mindful. It's a powerful trifecta of defense against temptation. And if you don't think one minute is enough, try it right now and see for yourself.

Don't cheat. Try your best to focus on your breaths. If your thoughts drift to the treat or anything else, and they probably will, gently bring them back to your breathing. It's been said before and it bears repeating that, even if you get distracted a lot while meditating, you're still benefiting. Just like anything else, you practice meditating to get better at it, not to do it perfectly on the first try.

2. Eat a healthier item. If it's a drink you're considering, I'd still recommend eating something healthy if you can. If no healthy food is available, then use #3 as your #2.

3. Do one push-up, one sit-up, dance for a minute, run in place for a minute, or do 15 jumping jacks. It's best to pick your preferred mini exercise now, rather than decide later. But the idea is to do something active. This can make you more mindful, more motivated to live a healthy lifestyle, and it could even cascade into a full workout. As with all mini habits, be open to doing more.

Just think of the times you engage in snack-eating. It's probably when you're relaxed, watching TV, and feeling a little bit lazy. Well, it's hard to feel lazy right after doing push-ups (or whatever your exercise choice may be)! It puts you in a much better mental state to resist or no longer desire the unhealthy food.

4. Drink a glass of water. We often mistake thirst for hunger. This would fix that!

5. Delay for 10 minutes. This is a great willpower strategy, as it takes much less willpower to delay an action than to resist it completely and doing so weakens your temptation. As Kelly McGonigal states in *The*

Willpower Instinct, "When the brain compares a cookie you have to wait ten minutes for to a longer-term reward, like losing weight, it no longer shows the same lopsided bias toward the sooner reward. It's the 'immediate' in immediate gratification that hijacks your brain and reverses your preferences."[169]

6. Distract yourself with a small step into another activity. It's good to have some alternate path ideas in mind before you're hit with temptation.

7. Present yourself with an alternate reward/bribe. This could be a TV show instead of nachos. It could be the decision to buy that T-shirt you've wanted instead of buying ice-cream. The idea is to choose a non-food reward that doesn't cause weight gain.

8. Take a walk. Just get out the front door and go. This is pretty fun to do, assuming you live in a safe neighborhood.

9. How was the walk? If you've come this far, this is already a MONSTER win! If you still want the item, but are high on these small victories and want one more, agree on a specific portion or agree to eat it another day, leaning toward the balance of shame-free (don't mindlessly indulge) and happy (never undercut yourself).

That concludes the temptation mini routine list. If you want to switch the order around, be my guest. Some might work better for you than others. Do not wait until you're tempted to decide which order the mini challenges are in, because making decisions depletes your willpower, which is an important resource to conserve (especially when tempted!).

Feel free to improvise if the situation calls for it. If your standard order is the one listed above, but you see a great alternate reward right away (#7 on the list), you can do that right away. That said, consistently doing the same mini challenges is helpful because, the more you do the same behaviors, the more habitual they will become when you're tempted. That's why I recommend having a go-to order of mini challenges that you can change on a case-by-case basis.

Craving Example

It's 11:34 PM, you're sitting on your couch, and "OMG I NEED ICE-CREAM NOW." This is a craving. Relax. Don't make it into a high-pressure "dieting decision." Don't fear caving into your craving. React as calmly as possible.

Realize that shame is the true enemy here, and that you can agree to two mini challenges to eat ice-cream without any shame. In the past, you'd let your desire for complete control translate into rigid rules and subsequent rebellion. Now, you're gently moving the behavior from all-or-nothing abstinence or bingeing into something that you calmly decide on.

1. Meditate for a minute
2. Eat a healthy alternative (or skip to #3 if unavailable)
3. Do one push-up (or alternate exercise)
4. Choose to continue with more challenges or go ahead and eat as much of it as you want. It's not forbidden, and nobody is going to stop you. As you eat it, however, don't turn your brain off. Be fully present, enjoy it, and think about how much of it you really want to eat, all things (including weight gain) considered.

The Law of Marginal Utility states that we'll enjoy our first slice of pizza more than our fifth slice. This is true for everything, which is why mindfulness is so important while eating. We've all likely eaten unhealthy food without even enjoying it, simply because we weren't being mindful. Whatever you eat, eat it mindfully.

When You Eat it, Make it Good
There will be times when you do your mini challenges (or not) and still consume the fried onion rings, the soda, or the fast food. It's fine. You're only human. When that time comes, do NOT try to cheat and trick your body with a "diet" treat.

Never, ever consume diet food. Not only are diet foods generally weight-gaining—because weight gain is a metabolic issue and they're worse for your metabolism than real sugar—but consuming "diet food" is one of the most psychologically backward things you can do if you're trying to lose weight.

It's the classic picture of the person bingeing on baked chips without worry. It's the person drinking diet soda after diet soda because, why not? They don't contain calories! It's the person guzzling down skim milk as if cows are going extinct. A "diet" product makes you believe that you're not going to gain weight by consuming it, or that you'll gain less weight than the "non-diet version." This isn't a reduction of shame, it's a reduction of truth! This belief is often wrong as it stands, but it becomes much worse when you feel compelled to consume *beyond* what you typically would consume because "it's diet."

When you consume unhealthy food, make sure it's full of real fat and real sugar. First, this food will actually be enjoyable and satisfying biologically, because your body can process these substances. Second, you'll be more conscious about your decision. It's the same reason why people recommend paying with cash instead of a credit card —when you hand over the cash, you feel the pain of losing it more than swiping a piece of plastic for hundreds of dollars. In the same way, when you chomp into that triple chocolate fudge sundae, you will feel the gain! Not shame, because you took care of that, but gain. It's good to associate these foods with weight gain, because that's the truth, even when they're pumped full of non-food chemicals and labeled "low-calorie" or "diet."

This isn't to make you feel bad about eating unhealthy food; it's to make you aware that there are no shortcuts to losing weight if you eat cake all day. Real food repairs your metabolic system by reducing inflammation, triggering proper reward and satiety responses, and giving the body time to heal itself from previous consumption of Frankenfoods.

Temptation Part 2: Stop Fighting Yourself

Even with the excellent strategies in this book, you will sabotage yourself if you approach your eating and movement habits with thoughts as innocent-sounding as, "I have to fight to eat well and do the best thing for my body." When you take a fighting stance against your current eating and movement habits, you're declaring war against your subconscious. Bad idea! Some people have struggled with the original *Mini Habits* system because they don't actually shed their old way of thinking.

Mini habits and the optional strategies in this book are strategically casual. A mini habit's strength is that it does NOT trigger any of these internal wars. Its strength is that it does NOT pose a threat to your current way of life. Like a taxi, it picks you up *where you are without judgment* and takes you someplace new.

The following is critical to understand, so reread it if necessary. If you ever feel resistance to doing a mini habit or going through the series of mini challenges when tempted, it's because *YOU are resisting* "the wrong way." It's because you are trying too hard to do "the right thing."

When you're tempted by something, your first instinct should not be, "Oh no, here's the craving. What can I do to stop this?" Even if your approach after that point is smart, your initial attitude of direct resistance to the temptation has already put you at a significant disadvantage.

I'm going to write this three times because it's that important.

The more you resist, the more you will feel resistance.
The more you resist, the more you will feel resistance.
The more you resist, the more you will feel resistance!

The way this works is that your resistance to "doing the wrong thing" riles up your subconscious (because it *wants* to do the wrong thing), and then you'll feel resistance to doing something as simple as one push-up or drinking a glass of water. On their own, these behaviors are laughably easy, but when you posture them as roadblocks to "the fun stuff," they're only slightly better than the massive goals people fail with on a regular basis.

The myth of the "quick fix" is one of the biggest hurdles to success with mini habits. Change your behavior through freedom, acceptance of where you are right now, and strategic and consistent movement toward better behaviors. It might be easiest to convey the right perspective in thoughts.

Good: "Those cookies look delicious and I want one. I know they're weight-gaining, so I'll go through two mini challenges and take it from there."
Bad: "Those cookies look delicious and I want one. Ugh. But I can't have one now! I shouldn't! I really want to lose this weight, but they look so good! I have to do something now! What strategies could I try to prevent myself from eating this?"

See how the first response is calm, collected, casual, and easy-going? See how the second response is frantic, defensive, and out of control? The first response works well because it doesn't create a win-lose scenario and it doesn't put any pressure on you to change yourself instantly. *It allows you to breathe.*

Also bad: "I'm going to do this mini challenge in order to defeat this craving."

The "end goal" of a mini habit is to do the mini habit. Nothing else. You can't expect a mini habit to save you from temptation, to turn into a full workout, or to make you love green beans on any given day. You *can* expect a mini habit to improve *any and all* of those areas over time. Does that make sense? If you ever place an in-the-moment expectation on a mini habit, you are no longer aiming for a mini habit, but for whatever your expectation is. The way to avoid this is to stop obsessing over individual events and results, and instead focus on being consistent with these small behaviors. In weight loss, every battle counts, but no single battle wins the war. Don't fear losing a battle; fear losing the war because you let a battle get the best of your emotions. (This goes back to the question "Is it worse to eat a cookie or to feel shame for eating a cookie?")

I understand that you *really* want to change. I understand that you *really* want to rid yourself of some of these bad habits that are keeping you from the health and body you desire. Funnel this energy into mastering this strategy and you will be rewarded with real progress, not the typical dieting rollercoaster of 10 pounds lost in 10 days followed by 15 pounds gained over the next 60 days.

The Emotional Cake Spiral

Food cravings for pleasurable foods are emotional and are largely driven by emotion. Pleasure eating triggers chemical reward signals that aren't present in hunger-driven eating.[170]

Knowing that food temptations are emotion-driven, consider this: What does the noble attempt to resist a food craving do to your emotional state? It increases the internal friction between your conscious and subconscious desires. This internal conflict *amplifies* your entire emotional state, which *increases* your subconscious desire to indulge.

1. You see the cake.
2. You want the cake.
3. You resist the cake at the thought of your weight loss goals.
4. You wrestle with the decision, intently resisting the cake (which increases the cake's mindshare).
5. You feel stressed out, exhausted, and willpower-depleted from the high-stakes decision.

6. Hey, that cake looks like the perfect distraction!
7. You eat the first bite of cake, its sweetness rewards your brain, and you immediately feel relief and relax. But soon after, a new wave of stress and shame overwhelm you. You lost the battle after fighting so hard, and now you feel worse than before.
8. As you feel more stress and shame, your desire for cake increases even more. Now you binge on the cake, because you feel like you've lost on so many levels and it doesn't matter anymore. You pretend that you don't care in that moment, but it's only because you can no longer handle the pain of losing the battle yet again and what that might mean for your future.

Has this process matched your experience? Do you see why we're taking a different approach?

You have a split second to decide how you will react when a food craving hits. If it's frantic and "Oh no! I mustn't!," then you're probably going to lose. Instead, take a deep breath, take your time, decide to be calm, and consider the strategic options in this book. If you want to try the optional temptation strategy, do it. If not, that's okay too.

Grocery Store Strategy: Healthy Swap

If you buy it, you will eat it.

The home eating war is won and lost in the grocery store. The food you buy creates your food environment at home, and it is very difficult to fight your environment if it is unfriendly to your goals.

If you only bought healthy food, you would eliminate your unhealthy snacking problem at home immediately and easily. I understand that it can get complicated with others in the same house who don't want to join you, but if that's the case, maybe you can ask them to hide their unhealthy snacks from you.

Here's the strategy I recommend while you're shopping: Buy groceries as usual. When you're ready to check out, remove one piece of unhealthy food and replace it with a healthy alternative. Why this way? It's awkward to tell you to buy at least one vegetable or one fruit. Unless your eating habits are exceptionally poor, you'll likely buy some amount of fruits and vegetables normally, and thus, an "at least one" requirement would do absolutely nothing for you. But replacing an unhealthy item you typically buy with a healthy substitute is an instant double win.

As with all mini habits, you can continue to make additional healthy replacements, but aim for just one to start. Here are a few examples:

- Exchange candy bars for no-sugar added or low-sugar dark chocolate
- Exchange ice-cream for bananas (freeze them and they taste like ice-cream) and/or other fruits
- Exchange regular spaghetti for spaghetti squash or whole wheat pasta
- Exchange spaghetti sauce for olive oil, pesto, and parmesan cheese
- Exchange white bread for whole grain bread (sprouted if possible)
- Exchange soda for sparkling or mineral water and 100% juice (and add only a little bit of juice to flavor the water)
- Exchange vegetable dip for hummus or guacamole (or, even better, ingredients to make your own!)
- Exchange salad dressing for olive oil and balsamic vinegar
- Exchange cereal and milk for yogurt and fruit (granola would be fine and is a better choice than cereal, but it's very hard to find any without added sweetener). Alternatively, plain steel-cut oats or plain rolled oats are decent options (steel-cut is better). Avoid the instant oatmeal packets loaded with sugar.
- Exchange meat for fish
- Exchange a processed snack for carrots, celery, radishes, cherry tomatoes, broccoli, or nuts (for snacking).

If you literally only buy processed foods, you can buy at least one kind of fresh or frozen vegetable (with some plan of how you'll consume it later; don't buy a squash and let it rot in your closet... don't put vegetables in your closet).

The Price of Healthy Food

People assume healthy eating is expensive, but is it really? Upfront, it is a bit more expensive. A meta-analysis of food costs covering 27 studies in 10 countries found that the difference in price between a healthy and

198

unhealthy diet was $1.50 per day per person.[171] That's $45 extra a month and $547 extra a year to make a significant positive investment in your health, weight, and well-being. It's a cliché but true to say that you'll save money by cutting down on medical costs when you eat healthy food and take care of yourself. The price of healthy food is less expensive than the long-term costs of eating unhealthy food.

Many people in the USA spend $5 or more every day on lattes and other superfluous foods and beverages. In fact, $1.50 is close to the price of getting a soda at a restaurant, and low-income people drink more sugary drinks than others.[172] It is possible for most to afford healthy food if it's prioritized.

Home Eating Strategy

The single best thing you can do for better home eating is to make healthy foods easily accessible. Accessibility plays a big role in your willingness to eat well. Buying healthy food is not the complete answer, because it's very easy to buy healthy food and let it spoil as you eat something else. There are three components to making healthy home eating more accessible.

1. Plan for consumption. When you buy broccoli, you should know how you're going to eat it. Be precise. Are you going to boil it in water? Are you going to sauté it in a pan? Are you going to use it for a casserole? Are you going to eat it raw, and will that include dip? Will it be a random snack food where you reach in the fridge and grab one or two, or a more robust snack of several stalks? Are you going to put it in a salad? You don't necessarily need to decide the exact use for it, but determine at least one or two ways you intend to eat it. This seed of intention can make a huge difference, and it will also prompt you to buy the right accessories you need while at the store. If you prefer to have broccoli in salads, but you don't have any lettuce, then you're much less likely to eat broccoli.

2. Learn faster ways to cook. If you're like me, you don't enjoy the time required to cook a decent meal. That said, there are plenty of fast ways to cook healthy food. One of my go-to methods is to stir-fry vegetables and meat. It takes 20-30 minutes max and afterwards I'll throw all cookware and dinnerware into the dishwasher. Easy. Rice cookers and slow cookers take longer, but they take about one minute of your time to prepare!

Salad is one of the healthiest things you can eat, and also one of the fastest to make, as it doesn't require any cooking. Sometimes I'll make simple salads with lettuce and just a couple other vegetables, olive oil, vinegar, pepper, all-purpose seasoning, and cheese. Other times, I'll create a mega salad with 15+ ingredients. The easiest way to do this is to cut a lot of vegetables in the first session. Cut an entire bunch of radishes, an entire stalk of celery, several whole carrots, a bell pepper, a few tomatoes, etc. Then use what you need for your salad, and store the rest in the refrigerator in sandwich bags or Tupperware. They'll last about 3-4 days, and the next time you want a salad, you can pull out all of your ingredients, throw them together in a bowl, and have a delicious mega salad in no time! For me, this sort of speed hack is the difference between me eating salads or eating at a restaurant.

3. Give yourself plenty of options. Do you have plenty of fruit for sweet cravings? Do you have healthy snacks like nuts or easily prepared fruits and vegetables? Do you have several viable healthy dinner options? Given that processed food is always going to be easier to prepare than healthy food, I rarely buy it (and I eat whatever I buy). But if I'm not buying processed food and I'm also not stocked with healthy food supplies, my only option is to eat out (and hope in vain that the restaurant uses quality ingredients).

To be satisfied with a healthy diet, which is absolutely possible, *you must have enough food*. You do need to balance this with the first component (plan for consumption), because the only thing worse than not having enough food around is having healthy food around and letting it spoil because you didn't plan how to consume it. That wastes your time, money, and motivation to eat healthy food.

The overarching goal is to create a home environment that is conducive to healthy living. Increase the ratio of healthy food to unhealthy food, plan for consumption, and learn what sort of food preparation you're willing to do. As much as I like to eat healthy food, I'm not willing to cook two hours every day to do it. If you are, that's great, but if you're not, then don't make that your win condition. Make it convenient, make it easy, and you'll do well.

Snacking Strategy

Emotional eating is a major cause of unnecessary snacking, and it is difficult to overcome. I know.

You might be expecting me to tell you that you need to get your emotions in check in order to fend off emotional eating. Not in this book. Mini habits are effective *because* they don't depend on emotional manipulation.

The smartest approach to overcoming emotions is indirect, because when you fight your emotions directly, well, you usually lose. Emotions are subconscious feelings that don't just go away because you want them to go away. In order to feel differently, you have to act differently. **Feeling itself is not a choice, but it is greatly affected by your choices.**

Every person hopefully learns at some point in their life that it works better to focus on things you can control. So, instead of trying to reverse the emotions that cause excess eating, we're going to rewire your emotional response software. Right now, you might be programmed to eat potato chips, ice-cream, and chocolate bars when you're stressed out or sad.

The Two Possible Emotional Support Systems

Being a human is hard work. I think we can all agree on that. Since life is hard, we tend to need support from others, and also from things.

Some people get their support from ice-cream, the couch, and a good TV show. This isn't even wrong in moderation. But if this is your *primary and regular* therapist in life, your body will almost surely accumulate fat.

You can get a similar type of support from things like going to the gym, eating healthy food, and meditating. Not only is this type of support more effective—because it strengthens rather than weakens your mind, body, and emotional fortitude long-term—but also these things can be done "excessively" without negative consequence. They're stackable!

When someone is faced with changing their behavior to achieve a result (weight loss), they may think about the enjoyable things they'll have to lose, and they should consider that. But they also need to consider what they're gaining. A balanced perspective is best.

The feeling I get after playing basketball for a couple of hours is one of the best feelings I know! I feel relaxed, worn out in a good way, satisfied from being active, and my endorphins are flowing. Exercise is proven to reduce stress and improve mood. Meditation does the same.

Matthieu Ricard credits meditation for his nickname, "The Happiest Man on Earth." Ricard is a Buddhist monk, and, in his TED Talk, he shared the results of a brain scan of his fellow monks. The monks were four standard deviations higher in left prefrontal cortex activity, the side of the brain associated with happiness. Their happiness by this measure was off the charts, because they meditate so much.[173] These sorts of activities can be a powerful defense against emotional eating, because they improve your underlying emotional health.

"Snackers Gonna Snack"
Snacking is fine. What's the problem? This isn't a starve-yourself diet. The same perspectives and ideologies apply to snacking as much as to dinner. Obviously, it's better for your weight to choose celery over cupcakes, but if you want to eat a snack because you're *hungry*, then it'd be foolish to restrict yourself, since weight is not lost (long-term) by eating less food, but by eating more healthy food.

Some people suggest that you only eat 3-5 meals per day without snacking. They don't understand what they ask of us snackers! Newsflash: It's possible to lose weight and snack at the same time. Forbidding snacking is a classic example of needless restriction that makes us rebel and grab a doughnut.

If you've decided to snack on something unhealthy, select the amount you want to consume and place it in a bowl. Don't select less than you want, as you'd be fighting the wrong battle there. If you go back and get more, that's fine if you really want it, but try to select how much you actually want next time. Studies have shown that "second helpings" result in more food consumed, compared to those who fill their plate to satisfaction at the first serving.

You're not artificially limiting your consumption by choosing your snack portion; you're avoiding the mindless "out of the bag" eating. If you're eating fruits or vegetables, take the whole bag and enjoy. Mindlessly eating food that helps you lose weight isn't such a problem, but be careful not to confuse raw fruits and vegetables with "fake healthy" options like organic vegetable chips or fruit cups with added sugar.

A good rule of thumb to follow is: Snack when hungry, not when bored. Snack because you need energy, not because you need a therapist. If you feel the desire to snack, and it isn't because you're hungry, you can take a look at the temptation mini challenge. The mini challenges can improve your mood and reduce or eliminate your craving if it's based on emotional distress.

Remember that the goal is not the strategy. The goal is to not choose ice-cream and cookies when you snack, or to not eat much of them if you do. The strategy is to *respect your craving*, not try to deprive yourself of it. Make calm, rational choices, such as going through the temptation mini challenges, choosing your portion size, eating mindfully, and stopping when you're satisfied. If you do this, you WILL eat less unhealthy food. Don't lose sight of this and begin falling back into the dieting mindset of "Oh no, I want chips. I need to resist it in order to succeed!" That's when you'll fail. Direct resistance is futile, and the goal is not the strategy. Don't forget it!

That said, your goal isn't to be ignored either. You should remain mindful of your goal to eat healthier food. If you stop caring about your goal and mindlessly go through the motions of the strategies in this book, then you'll struggle to do the right thing. Be mindful of your goal *and* strategic with your actions—that's what you need to succeed.

Eating Out Strategy

In most cases, it's hard to lose weight when you eat out frequently. Eating out is one of my favorite things to do and I do it often, but I'm very selective of where and what I eat. When you eat at a restaurant, you can't assume that their food is healthy, as it likely has unhealthy additives and unnecessary amounts of sugar, sodium, and fat. Restaurant food is generally made for taste, not health, especially since customers are oblivious to the ingredients used (something I find frustrating).

It's unusual for customers to ask about ingredients and nutrition information. This made sense back when food was simple, but now it's more important than ever to know what you're eating, and a restaurant is one of the few places where you may have to "eat blindly."

Assume that restaurant ingredients are unhealthy unless the food is obviously simple (like steamed vegetables) or the restaurant explicitly says what ingredients they do (and don't) use. More restaurants these days are advertising about things like no artificial colors or flavors, no preservatives, antibiotic free meat, and so on. Just be warned that the meal probably still has excessive sugar, salt, and fat.

Check the Ingredients

When you are thinking about eating at a restaurant, I recommend Googling "[restaurant name] ingredients" first. Not many restaurants list their ingredients online, but some major chains do. If you don't find exact ingredients, you might find some kind of commentary about them. If you find the ingredient list and don't recognize an ingredient, it's probably some chemically made preservative or flavor enhancer. If the ingredient list is extremely long, that's also a warning sign.

Caring about your weight means caring about the ingredients in your food. It would be easier if good ingredients were standard, but they are more expensive, and consumers rarely ask about ingredients. As businesses, restaurants have a much greater incentive to use cheap ingredients that taste great.

Far more important than how often you eat out is:

1.   Where you eat
2.   What you order

In general, healthy meals are simple dishes of vegetables (and meat if you're not vegetarian), and the worst dishes contain fried foods, oils, and sauces (sauces are the hidden weight gainer in many restaurants). Sauces and dressings taste great, but they almost always contain a massive amount of unhealthy fat (soybean oil), sugar, and chemical additives, and they're not satiating.

The more aware you are about restaurant food, the better you'll be able to manage your eating out frequency and choices. Do some research on your favorite restaurants to investigate their food quality. In addition to checking out the ingredients, you can usually find restaurant menus online to see if there are any healthy options that appeal to you.

Ask the Right Questions

If you're considering a dish with meat or fish, ask how they cook it. Look to get it broiled, baked, or grilled. On several occasions, I've accidentally ordered fried food, because the menu didn't specify the cooking method used and I didn't ask. Now I ask if it doesn't say.

Of course, none of these are *rules*—you can eat whatever you want. There's a difference between knowing the right way and feeling pressured to live it perfectly. These details are important to be aware of because of how easy it is to mistake an unhealthy meal for a healthy one when eating out. The worst thing is thinking you're eating healthy food when you're not!

Mindset check: Eating high quality food isn't "required suffering" or "punishment" for people who want to lose weight. What you just read is exactly how I approach restaurant eating and I'm not overweight—I just care about my health. I'll eat at places without checking ingredients sometimes, but I know the ingredients of the restaurants I eat at regularly. It's what you do most often that defines your long-term results.

Peer Pressure Strategy

The Unseen Power of a Hot Dog

When I was a kid, I ate by taste (remember, I ate chapstick because I liked the flavor). If I still operated by that program, I would love eating hot dogs. But when I look at a hot dog, I see that processed bun full of preservatives, and when I look at the hot dog meat, I think of the disgusting ingredients inside.

It's not common to talk about food ingredients in many cultures. In the United States, some guy would say, "It's just a hot dog, dude." It's unusual to not want to ingest a lab abomination that isn't fit for human consumption. And why? Anecdotes abound, such as "My uncle ate a hot dog every day and he lived until he was 88," which says much more about the uncle's vitality than the hot dog's suitability for consumption. Association is also at play, this time to our detriment. Many people have their fondest memories associated with the worst foods. Baseball games in America are associated with hot dogs. Movies at the theater are associated with bathtub-sized soft drinks and a bucket of salty butter sprinkled with a few pieces of popcorn. Memorable parties and holiday gatherings are almost explicitly comprised of unhealthy foods.

These associations have *layers* of influence on us—personal memories on top of societal pairings (hot dogs and baseball, cakes and birthdays, etc.), on top of current social norms (getting beers with the guys, eating pizza at college, etc.). These social forces are the most potent influencers in the world, and they're making us fatter.

If I were to bring up the non-food-like qualities of a hot dog, I could potentially even *offend* someone. Maybe this someone grew up going to baseball games with his father, and always got a hot dog. The father's since passed away, and now the hot dog is a part of his memory, so by telling him how terrible hot dogs are, he sees it as alleging that his dad was a bad father because he let his son eat hot dogs, or that I'm judging *him* because he eats hot dogs. That's why food is not just a discussion about calories, nutrition, and food quality. It's also culture, society, memories, emotions, habits, and experiences. The quality of food is the surface-level discussion that dominates weight loss books. But it's all of that other stuff in our subconscious that has the greatest influence on what we eat.

Different Results Require Being Different
A 2016 study found that only 2.7% of Americans matched four healthy lifestyle characteristics (non-smoking, healthy body fat percentage, active lifestyle, and healthy diet). That should surprise no one. It's weird not to drink socially when you go out, to suggest vegetables as a snack, or to order a big salad. That's because sadly it isn't normal to eat real food anymore.

To be at a healthy weight, you have to be different from the average person, because the average person in many countries today is overweight. Some people get this concept right, but with the wrong applications. They switch to diet foods and drinks, try to starve themselves, and do "cleanses." It's estimated that 45 million Americans diet every year, and very few succeed. You don't just want different results from the overweight population; you also want different results from the *dieting* population. *That means you have to approach this differently from almost everyone around you (the mini habits approach is different and it works).*

Even with Better Information, Behavior Change Lags
Nutritional information has gotten better recently, and many people are trying to change. For example, soda consumption hit a 30-year low in

2015, with diet soda seeing the steepest decline (hooray!).[174] That is to say that all hope is not lost, and some of us are waking up to the processed food experiment that's gone horribly wrong.

Still, even as nutrition education increases and people know what they should do, *lasting behavior change remains a rarity*. It's estimated that 25% of Americans eat fast food every day. In America, fast food revenue surpassed $200 billion in 2015. Worldwide, it was $570 billion. That's billion with a "B."

That's why this book is a game changer. These strategies are so powerful that they can empower you to swim against this worldwide current of obesity.

Peer Pressure Strategy

Now that we've covered just how much pressure there is against healthy living (a lot), here's what to do about it. First of all, if any of your friendships *depend* on you living an unhealthy lifestyle, then that's an unhealthy friendship by definition! Real friends won't judge you or try to make you feel bad for making good decisions. You should be able to remain friends with people as you gradually shift your behavior with mini habits, but be aware that any lifestyle change—even when done gradually —can alter the dynamic of your relationships.

For each food decision that is being influenced by your peers, ask yourself what's more important to you at the moment—your health or conforming to your surroundings. I don't mean that in a demeaning way, and I'm not implying that you "should always choose your health." There are times when we would rather join the group than choose the healthier option, and there's nothing wrong with it. The problem is when you have no control over that decision and peer pressure wins out every time. If you have a track record of caving to peer pressure, you need to practice being more independent with your choices. Your peers don't have to live with your choices, only you do. Here are some ways to navigate the peer pressure minefield.

Speak from preference, not from obligation. People almost always respect preference. If you don't want something, people aren't going to pressure you too much into eating it. But if you "can't have it" because you're "on a diet," then they might see if they can coax you into indulging. One reason why people want you to join them in indulgence, by the way, is so they'll feel better about their unhealthy lifestyle choices.

If you order a salad and everyone else gets fried chicken and fries, your salad may make the others question their decision (or feel bad about it). It's as if the lettuce in your bowl lectures them as they try to enjoy their fried food.

Let's say that you've decided to choose the healthier option despite your friends indulging. Bravo! But one of your friends makes a comment or a question about your choice (expect this, because healthy eating is unusual). What do you say?

The worst thing you can do is act as if skipping the chocolate cake isn't actually your choice. This is an appeal to authority in order to reduce your responsibility for the decision. It seems as if it gets you out of questioning because you're "just following instructions," but this often incites the wrong response from others. If I'm your friend and you tell me that you "can't have it" because of some phantom authority you've made up, I might be motivated to set you free from that authority who isn't allowing you to enjoy life. You've implied that you want the cake but have no freedom of choice. You might start thinking about fighting back against this phantom authority too. Nobody likes the fun police!

If you confidently say that you don't want chocolate cake, then your friends have very little incentive to argue with you. Your personal preference is the ultimate authority when it comes to your food choices, and most people intuitively understand and respect that. If someone presses you on it, simply continue to state what you want (or don't want). It's that simple. You don't need any "I'm on a diet" excuses to not eat dessert. There are plenty of other reasons to not eat dessert that can come from *you*.

Correct and strong responses
"I don't want [unhealthy food]."
"I really want [healthy food]."
"I'd rather have [healthy food] than [unhealthy food]."

Weak responses
"I can't eat [unhealthy food], I'm on a diet."
"No thanks. I'm watching my weight."
"I have to eat this [healthy food]."

Don't impose your healthy choices on others, either. One of the best things you can do when eating healthy food is to make it clear that you're not judging anyone else for their food choices (nor should you!). What people choose to eat is personal, amoral, and should concern nobody else. If someone remarks about how healthy my meal looks, it might be because they feel shameful about their meal choice, so I'll often compliment their meal or mention that I also eat what they ordered sometimes. And it's true. As I've said, I've eaten all of the worst foods, just as most people have. To judge someone on what they eat in a single meal is nonsensical and unproductive.

If you want to encourage others to eat more healthily, piling on the guilt is not the way. Nobody enjoys the healthy food police. Even encouraging someone to eat healthier food with good intentions can imply there's guilt involved. It's a sensitive subject for many, so be careful out there! The best way to handle it is exactly the way you'll be thinking about food with *Mini Habits for Weight Loss*—food choices aren't ever bad, wrong, forbidden, or illegal.

Some food is terrible for our health and weight, but we have every right to choose to eat it. If that's what you take away from this book and you decide that you just want to eat cake in bed all day and not feel bad about it, that's your choice, and I don't judge you for it. The path to lasting success is through freedom, choice, empowerment, and mindfulness, not guilt and shame.

In conclusion, the way to navigate peer pressure is through mutual respect. Demand respect for your food choices and desires, and give the same respect to others in return.

Parties and Holidays Strategy

The holidays are a big deal, not just in life, but for weight loss. A Texas Tech study found that Americans gain about 1.5 pounds over the six-week holiday season, which is about 75% of the entire year's average weight gain.[175] Two pounds a year sounds small, but over 20 years, that's 40 extra pounds.

Thus, the seemingly small weight gain during the holidays is devastating to long-term weight loss plans. Your behavior at holiday (and other) parties is important, because these are the situations where you're most likely to make poor decisions due to terrible food options, peer pressure, and the "special occasion" effect.

Party Snack Psychology

Imagine you're at a party with loads of snacks, some healthy and some unhealthy. (If you find *any* healthy snacks at a party, you're probably the one who brought them.) When looking at the vegetables and cookies, don't think in all-or-nothing terms, which leads to rebellion. It's not vegetables or cookies—think about how best to merge your sweet tooth with your healthy goals, and do your best to "lean healthy." The difference between a person who eats healthy and one who eats poorly is smaller than you think. One leans healthy and the other leans unhealthy. One gains a pound over the holidays and the other gains none or loses a little bit of weight each month, including during the holidays. Small choices accumulate into big changes over time.

Holidays are special occasions, not special food occasions. Food is not what makes the holidays special. Or, rather, it shouldn't be. Otherwise, the holidays are no different from a trip to a nice buffet.

Do your best to dissociate holiday cheer with food and beer. This isn't to say you mustn't eat anything unhealthy; it's to remind you not to give up responsibility for your food choices because "Oh, it's the holidays, and therefore I can eat mindlessly!" If you really begin to change—and your daily mini habits will help you do that—your healthy lifestyle won't last 46 weeks per year but all year. Therefore, the holidays are a good indicator of where you *really* stand. Dieters feel as if they're being torn apart every holiday season because they know what they "should" do, but they don't want to do it. People who change their subconscious preferences no longer desire these foods to the extent they once did.

It's hard to try to convey the mindfulness and consistency needed for success without giving that "You can't have fun anymore" vibe. I'm aware that dieting has made all of us prone to assume the "I can't do XYZ because ____" mindset. That's a failing plan. Real change means you don't *want* to do XYZ.

Party Strategy

This is not a situation in which you "need to be careful" and "watch out." That gives the wrong connotation, and you'll be right back to your dieting ways of direct resistance. Be calmly strategic at parties. Negotiate with yourself and make deals. *Be mindful.* For example, maybe you negotiate to have some candy, but drink water, or you choose to drink booze, but snack on carrots and celery. It's all delicious. You're calm. You win.

As you think about these decisions on what foods to eat and how much, one of the best underlying and decision-driving mindsets is to simply care about your body and your health. That alone can make you genuinely not want some of the food that isn't worth the cost. The reason I don't eat much candy is because I know (and don't like the thought of) the effect it has on my body. There may be some foods—triple fudge cake—that you think *are* worth the cost, and, in that case, maybe you take a slice and eat it slowly, mindfully, and without shame.

When eating a slice of triple fudge cake, there are a few ways to go about it.

1. Rushed, frantic, stressed, and triggered eating, in which you resist it until the last second, when you cave and shove it into your mouth. The relief you feel is as much about the resistance battle being over as it is the sugar and taste of the cake.
2. Eating it normally, but with crippling thoughts of shame and failure.
3. Not eating it and feeling completely deprived of all joy and life.
4. Eating a slice slowly, mindfully, and joyfully, enjoying every bite shamelessly, and being mindful of when you're satisfied enough to stop eating it (even if you haven't finished what's on your plate).

Never forget that the enemy of weight loss is processed food, but the enemy of behavior change for weight loss (what counts the most) is some combination of mindless eating, shame, inconsistency, and giving up.

What Mindfulness Looks Like
- When you don't want to eat something unhealthy, you won't.
- When you only "sort of" want to eat something unhealthy, you'll wait until you want to eat it.
- When you eat something unhealthy, you'll savor every bite and enjoy it more than anyone else.

What No Shame Eating Looks Like
- When you eat something unhealthy, you'll be far less likely to binge.
- After you eat something unhealthy, it won't affect your next

decision (which is good).

- After you eat something unhealthy, you will remain strong and confident in your weight loss journey, not crippled and devastated.

What Consistency Looks Like

- When you eat healthy food consistently, the occasional unhealthy food has no impact on your success.
- When you act in a new way consistently, you will form a habit and begin to prefer that behavior.
- When you win consistently, you will expect to win and act like a winner.

What Never Giving up Does

Those who never give up will find their way to success. Persistence is the common factor in every success story. Just because you have success every day with your mini habits does not mean that you won't have off days. It's key to mitigate the psychological damage from such days, and that's done by combining the above factors with the decision to never give up.

By going into parties with a calm, strategic mindset, you'll be one of the few people there who can have fun and make progress. Over time, you'll make better choices, which will lead to healthier preferences.

10

Conclusion

You've Tried Dieting Many Times, Try This Once

"All men can see these tactics whereby I conquer, but what none can see is the strategy out of which victory is evolved."
~ Sun Tzu

New Mindset

I used one push-up per day to become a frequent exerciser. It prioritized consistency in order to change the brain and familiarize it with exercise, increased short- and long-term motivation with early success, maximized momentum-based progress by starting the process of exercising every day, and improved my morale by ensuring a long winning streak. Those who see the one push-up tactic may compare it to something like the "100 push-up challenge," which is to do 100 push-ups per day. Comparing these tactics without considering their underlying strategy often leads to the wrong choice. The strategy behind 100 push-ups a day is comparatively weak. The idea is to create rapid progress and snowball motivation, but it's almost always thwarted by the slow-change nature of the brain, fickle motivation, limited willpower, and the unpredictability of life.

Most people who want to lose weight adopt some form of dieting as their tactic of choice. The strategy behind dieting is to lose weight by doing something more extreme than the people not trying to lose weight (one such tactic is intentionally creating a calorie deficit). This sort of change is counteracted biologically and neurologically in ways beyond our control. So even if you succeed with this plan, you're likely to fail with your goal, as shown in the introduction. That's how terrible the strategy is—when executed perfectly, it fails. Not only are extreme changes not necessary to lose weight, they are also counterproductive.

The new mindset we've discussed is recognizing that weight loss and behavior change are best done gradually. When change is gradual, we don't trigger the brain's countermeasures that make us revert to old habits or the body's countermeasures that make us regain the weight (and then some). Instead, we will methodically shift the baseline fat set point lower and lower as we change our behavioral and dietary preferences (which are dictated by habit).

To go along with this, we've clarified that weight loss is not a matter of carbs, fat, or calories, but of food quality. To isolate any of those factors would be an incorrect, albeit popular, oversimplification. There are different *types* of each macronutrient, and they have vastly different effects in the body. Olive oil and coconut oil are healthy fats. Trans fats and vegetable oils are unhealthy fats. Fruits and vegetables are healthy carbs. Ultra-processed foods like chips, soda crackers, and fries are unhealthy carbs. Anyone can point to an example of an unhealthy fat or an unhealthy carb and say, "That's it! It's the carbs (or fat)!" This is like meeting one mean person and concluding that all people are mean. Some of us are nice! Observational science consistently finds that fats, carbs, and calories are sometimes good and sometimes bad, depending on the quality of the source.

Some people say that we're just eating too much food. That may be true, but if so, *why* are we eating too much food? Were our ancestors more adept at counting calories or buying sugar-free cupcakes? The factors that really matter are satiety, satisfaction, micronutrients, and phytonutrients. If you have two foods that are 100 calories, but one is 14 times heavier and more filling per calorie, how can you say that calories are all that matter? Strawberries are 14 times heavier per calorie than potato chips. To anyone who still believes in calorie counting, I invite you to put it to the test with the strawberry chips challenge!

The Strawberry Chips Challenge

Take this challenge at your own risk. I don't recommend it.

One day, see how far you can get eating one 8-ounce bag of potato chips. I imagine I could eat the entire bag in one sitting. Another day, see how far you can get eating 7.2 pounds of strawberries. One bag of chips and 7.2 pounds of strawberries contain the same amount of calories, so as long as you "count them," it doesn't matter if you eat chips or strawberries, right? Oh, what's that? Your stomach exploded when you tried to eat seven pounds of strawberries? Disclaimer: *Do not try this challenge at home... or anywhere else.*

If anyone ever suggests to you that counting calories is all that matters, tell them to take this challenge. When they refuse or give an excuse like, "Well, you just have to eat the chips in moderation," then you can clarify to them that satiety-per-calorie matters more than just calories (and so does micro-nutrition, but that's less tangible than seven pounds of strawberries, so we'll keep it simple). If you count calories, you risk being hungry and wrecking your metabolism. Eat healthy foods that satisfy your hunger and nutritional needs. That's the right solution.

To summarize the new mindset of this book: Don't worry about carbs, fats, protein, and calories. Only concern yourself with the quality of food you're eating. If you eat quality food, all of those other things will fall into place. It's not easy to eat quality food in a world obsessed with processed food, but it's easier than counting calories, carbs, or fat. No math necessary. I like math, but not calorie counting math.

The 8 Sacred Laws of Mini Habits for Weight Loss

Do not break these laws. If you do, you will greatly reduce your chance of success.

1. No Dieting
Do not diet and call it mini habits. Mini habits are small and easy changes, not, "Sorry, I can't eat that. I'm watching my weight and can only eat salad." Dieting forces you to eat healthy food, but your mini habits will gently teach you to enjoy it more.

2. No Limits on Unhealthy Food, No Deprivation
Your body is used to a certain way of eating, and, if you threaten that, you will lose 95% of the time (this is the failure rate of dieting, according to some studies). If you feel a powerful craving to eat a burger, think about it and apply the optional temptation strategy in this book to see if it changes, but if it's still there and strong, YOU HAD BETTER EAT THAT BURGER! Enjoy it, too.

If your cravings frustrate you because you want to make progress, you still can make progress. Chew each bite 30 times. Drink water. See if a lettuce wrap would be agreeable instead of the bun. There are battles within the battle, and the optimal decision is not usually at the extreme. Even if you lose the entire battle, it is less important than winning the war. We don't swing blindly anymore. We choose fights we know we can win. Patience and cunning strategy lead to victory.

The way to eat less junk food is to allow it unconditionally, and to employ strategies to help you make healthier decisions. Leave deprivation to the dieters. If you ever feel deprived while following the *Mini Habits for Weight Loss* strategy, either you're doing it wrong, or you need to tweak it to your needs.

This doesn't mean you should always eat unhealthy food if you crave it. If you prefer a burger, but find salmon and vegetables to be almost as desirable, then go ahead and get the salmon. That's not deprivation of an uncontrollable craving; it's the better choice between two desirable options.

3. Feel No Shame

There's no reason to feel shameful about what you weigh or what you eat. If you just ate a slice of pizza in two bites, you didn't commit a crime, you didn't destroy your chance at losing weight, and you certainly didn't do anything "wrong." Food is amoral. That is, there is no morality associated with food (except with certain religions—you know who you are).

That is to say that consuming burgers, sodas, fries, candy, Brussels sprouts, French onion soup, or bacon should have no effect on how you feel about yourself. Think about it—nearly everyone has eaten nearly every type of food. Why should *you* feel bad about eating a food everyone else has eaten before? It doesn't make sense. I'm a health nut, but I've consumed all of the very worst processed food. In the 1990s there was a briefly popular soft drink called Surge, and I drank it as if I thought it gave me superpowers. Surge had more sugar and caffeine than most soft drinks, so it felt like a superpower at times.

Food is how we survive. It's enjoyable, except for the cricket I ate in Thailand. That fried food your neighbors just ate still gave them life-sustaining energy.

You can be fully aware of how food impacts your body without feeling shame for eating it. By not being on a diet, you'll have a much easier time with this, but you might have to remind yourself if your old "dieting" instinct kicks in. You might even need to purposefully and confidently eat unhealthy food to prove to yourself that it's not criminal. You have a plan to lose weight, but it's nothing like the ones that didn't work. It's rooted in your personal freedom, autonomy, and empowerment. No foods are restricted.

Make the decision right now to drop all shame about your weight and the foods you eat. You will feel 100 pounds lighter just from shedding shame, and you sure won't miss it!

4. Be the Captain, Not the Deckhand

This one is important. Many people, when reading a strategy-driven book, will attempt to "follow the steps to success." For this strategy especially, you have to take initiative. Be the leader, and use this as a guidebook for *your* change. All of the best leaders have advisors. This book is your advisor, but you're the one calling the shots. This is your life.

If, instead, you demote yourself to a deckhand, you'll be following literal directions and you may miss the *concepts* that make this strategy effective. Those who have the greatest success with this strategy will be the ones who "get it." They'll see the concepts at play, such as how small, imperceptible changes won't trigger the body or the subconscious into countermeasures, how shame destroys us while small wins encourage us, how autonomy empowers us to new heights while rules beat us down until we rebel, or how consistency matters more than anything else because it shapes our habitual preferences.

One of the best ways to describe the difference between the captain and the deckhand is this: The captain will make changes as necessary, while the deckhand will only do what he's told. The captain will be more aggressive in general, making bonus reps a more likely occurrence (and bonus reps are one of the most exciting aspects of this strategy).

You're free to live as you wish, but you'll be armed with potent strategies to change yourself for the better. This is a lifelong strategy, because you aren't giving up your freedom. You're adding power to your life, not following directions and depriving yourself to get a result. Please take the wheel, Captain. (May I suggest Hawaii?)

5. Never Stop Self-Negotiating and Strategizing (Don't Allow Complete Rebellion)

The moment you say, "screw it" and binge is the moment you've lost, not because you're about to eat an entire cheesecake, but because you've let the "strict" side of you—the one that wants to lose weight—domineer over your carnal, cheesecake-loving self for too long. In order for this venture to be a success, you have to be happy with your decisions consciously *and* subconsciously. You need to make decisions that at once support a healthier you and provide you with the carnal comfort you need.

Counterintuitively, the way to stop rebellion is not through brute force tactics (like willpower), but to make rebellion seem like a ridiculous idea.

People don't rebel against things they like. Make sure you like what you're doing. This strategy is built to be very agreeable, but feel free to customize it to better meet your needs. Just be careful not to "customize it" into a typical dieting system of rules and restrictions. That's why understanding these concepts is critical to success.

6. Rely on Your Healthy Heroes

Take note of healthy foods that you like. These are your heroes, and you can rely on them to carry you. If you don't like vegetables much, but you have an unusual affinity for broccoli, eat lots of broccoli. If you like to snack on radishes, do it often. If you love the taste of asparagus, always have it on hand.

Those who diet tend to force-eat food they don't enjoy. Some food is an acquired taste, so it's not a bad idea to make yourself eat food you don't enjoy on occasion, but don't make it your primary strategy. You can avoid the "suffer for weight loss" mindset by choosing food you like. If you don't think you like any healthy food, then continue to experiment. You haven't tried all of it, and you're most likely comparing it to processed food. When you eat lots of processed food, healthy food won't seem as appealing because it's different. Don't think of eating healthy food as substitution; think of it as practice. The more consistently you eat healthy food, the more you'll want it.

7. Try

Mini habits are powerful little behaviors. They can change your life. They are not, however, magic. I mean, they're *almost magical* in how well they work, but you can't think, "Okay, I did one push-up and nothing happened." Underlying that quote is someone who is *indifferent to success, hoping to get it without trying.* In order to make the mini habits strategy work, you still have to try, just as you would with any other strategy. The total effort required for success with mini habits is lower than most, but effort is still required.

8. Never Mistake Your Goal for Your Strategy, and Use Them Both Properly

Your goal is where you'd like to go. Your strategy is how you plan to get there.

Processed food is terrible. It is the bane of weight loss. Therefore, the goal is to stop eating it. The best strategy, however, is not to "stop eating it," since a "junk food ban" will make you feel deprived when you don't eat it and shameful when you do.

Your goal is not your strategy, but your goal is still important. Just as bad as using the goal as your strategy is ignoring the goal and mindlessly using the strategy. If you eat a carrot and passively wait for something to happen because "the strategy is supposed to work," then you're not thinking about your original goal, which is to live healthier.

When you know your goals and you use smart strategies to achieve them, you will thrive. Your goals give you direction and desire, and your strategy puts you in the best position to reach the goal. Here are a couple of examples.

Mistake (using your goal as your strategy): "I want to stop drinking soda, therefore I'll stop drinking soda."
Correct: "I want to stop drinking soda. My strategy is to allow myself to drink it, but stock up with several healthy alternatives, and every time I'm tempted to drink soda, I'll go through the mini obstacle course I've set up, including drinking a glass of refreshing lime-infused water."

Mistake (ignoring the goal and mindlessly trying the strategy): "I'll eat one carrot at 3 PM every day because Stephen said." (This *could* work, but it's not the ideal perspective.)
Correct: "I want to lose weight by eating more vegetables. My strategy for that is to eat one carrot at 3 PM every day to decrease my resistance to eating vegetables over time. Also, I can use that momentum on some days to eat more carrots or other vegetables in that moment, or maybe it will encourage me to keep making good decisions for the rest of the day. The first small step should break through the resistance I usually feel and put me on the right track, while doing it every day could develop the carrot-eating habit."

Mini Habits for Weight Loss Strategy Recap

Since we've covered so much information, you might be wondering how to put it all together. Let's take a zoomed-out look at the entire actionable portion of the book.

The *Mini Habits for Weight Loss* strategy has four components. Three of these are optional, and one is a daily requirement. We've covered these in detail, and this is the overview of how they all work together.

Daily Mini Habits (mandatory): Choose 1-4 mini habits you'll do every day, and select an implementation plan that suits your personality and lifestyle (as covered in the "Mini Habit Plans" section). These daily mini habits are the most important component for change, because they're your "base" of consistent progress. They're easy to do, even on a bad day, which is why remarkable consistency is not just possible but highly probable. Daily mini habits are the *only* mandatory aspect of the entire mini habits strategy. You must do these every day if you want to succeed. Since these are a "must-do" requirement, it's helpful to remind yourself just how *easy* these behaviors are, or else you might feel controlled and rebel. If you feel resistance to your mini habits, consider these tips:

1. Imagine how easy it would be to actually perform your small goal. Visualize it.
2. Don't compare your goal to other tasks.
3. Be eager for any amount of forward motion.
4. Set the precedent of ignoring your circumstances. Progress is rarely convenient.
5. Never underestimate what a small good decision can do for your life in the short term and long term.

If you can internalize that mindset, you will thrive. Beyond mini habits, the rest of the strategy is about shifting your mindset and making use of the following optional strategies to help you.

Temptation Strategy (optional): Within the "Situational Strategies" chapter is a broad temptation strategy that umbrellas over all situations. The temptation strategy is designed to reduce shame, decrease the severity of your cravings, and empower you to make better decisions now and later. These three things are accomplished through a simple "mini obstacle course." This strategy is smart because it strengthens you even when you "lose" and indulge in a craving. You're not going to resist processed food perfectly for the rest of your life, so any strategy that counts on your doing that (read: every other weight loss book you've ever read) is a poor one.

The temptation strategy is optional, meaning you do *not* have to try to implement it every time you're tempted. Your goal is to make healthier choices, and this is a tool to help you accomplish that. If I suggested that you make it mandatory, it would interfere with the broader mini habits strategy. If you required yourself to use this strategy every time you're tempted but you didn't always do it, then you might think you're failing or that the mini habits strategy isn't working as a whole and stop doing your daily mini habits. This is obviously something to avoid, since the daily mini habits are most important, and this is more of a bonus if you can do it.

That said, this is a very powerful strategy that I recommend you do as often as possible. But don't ever feel like you've failed or that you've "messed up" if you are tempted by food and just eat it without trying this. This is optional, but I would prioritize it over the other optional strategies, since cravings and temptation play such a large role in eating.

Situational Strategies (optional): Life presents you with plenty of challenges if you want to lose weight. You'll find yourself in situations in which it's difficult to make healthy decisions. Most people try to use willpower to mitigate all of these situations, and it works well... until it fails. Since willpower does fail us sometimes, it's better to use strategies that are effective in any willpower or motivational state.

In the "Situational Strategies" chapter, we covered general temptation, six other common situations, and the ideal strategy for each one. You can use them as a reference. For example, when you're about to attend a party, you can review the "Parties and Holidays" strategy guide. Having different strategies for different situations is more customized than dieting, which ignores the reality of life and gives you a confining "no matter what" ultimatum.

Mini Challenges (optional): You can choose to do these fun and easy challenges on a case-by-case basis. These are like the situational strategies, but they involve movement instead of eating.

If you want, you can try making one of these into a standard mini habit if it's attached to something you do every day. For example, if you watch TV every day, then you can implement the "TV Challenge" or the "TV Commercial Challenge" as a daily requirement. This is more difficult than a typical mini habit, because it can be triggered several times per day. If you watch three hours of TV, that might be 24 commercial breaks, which would mean you're getting up and moving 24 times per day. That's quite a lot to do on every day. It's doable and easy in each individual case, but to have to do it *that many times* can be intimidating. That's why I recommend these as optional in most cases.

If you have a stairs vs. elevator choice every day, maybe at your workplace, then you could make that into a mini habit by choosing one specific cue. Maybe you will decide to use the stairs as you go into and/or leave work, but use the elevator at lunch. Likewise, maybe you'll choose to do a mini exercise routine before watching TV, but not during commercials. Whether or not you make these mandatory depends on how frequently you run into this situation, and your overall "mini habits load." It's *not* a good thing to have too many mini habits.

Be sure to manage your daily requirements and optional activities into something that's comfortable. Your plan can challenge you *slightly*, but daily success matters more than "challenging yourself," because it forms habits, and habits allow you to challenge yourself more often and in greater intensity without risk of total failure.

Habits set the floor for your worst days. For example, my worst writing day technically has a floor of 50 words. That's just on paper as my mini habit. Since I've had this mini habit for more than two years and my writing habit is strong, my *worst* days are more like 1,000 words written. Others—including me before mini habits—start out aiming for something challenging like 1,000 words per day, and often fail to hit that mark or quit from burnout. Because I aimed for consistency and built the writing habit, writing 1,000 words a day is now an average or below-average day for me, when it used to be "an extraordinary accomplishment." This is the power of habit, and don't forget it.

The fun thing about these mini challenges (and also your daily mini habits) is that, whenever you take a small positive action, you'll feel good about yourself. I can't overstate how crucial this is to your success. When I take the stairs instead of the elevator in my apartment, I feel disproportionately good about myself. Someone should slap me and say, "Dude, you just went up some stairs. Calm down." It sounds silly, but you'll see what I mean. It's addictive and rewarding to accumulate these small wins, which is what this whole strategy is based on doing.

Final Words

You are now armed with strategies that can take you the distance. You will be able to apply these strategies seven years from now as well as today, because they are designed for lifelong use and success. If you've tried the frantic, motivation-driven push to lose weight quickly, you know how that ends. If you've tried to change your diet overnight, you know how that ends. Try this way, and you'll see a different, happier ending.

To make real, lasting progress, you need to make changes you can sustain. And these changes are not going to become more difficult over time, but easier to do as your brain familiarizes with them. When they finally become habitual, they will be your new *preferences*, and then you won't have to operate under any plan. You'll just be living your new lifestyle.

Lasting weight loss is possible, not through dieting, but through small and consistent changes that mesh with the way your body and brain prefer to change. If a behavior is "too small to fail" and so easy that you can do it on your worst day, what can stop you from doing it? Nothing, and that means that nothing will stop you from changing your behavior and getting healthier.

Mini Habits for Weight Loss is success- and practice-driven. Too many people set goals they can't reach. That isn't fruitful. We get better by practicing hitting targets, not by failing to hit targets out of our reach. Imagine succeeding every day, not just when you're motivated. Imagine growing in confidence every day. Imagine losing weight over the next year without having fear of regaining it because of how you've changed from the inside out, rather than from forced, conscious-only, willpower-draining, outside-in dieting programs.

This is your chance to try a weight loss strategy that can actually work long-term. I hope you take advantage of the opportunity before you. As the saying goes, once you go mini, you don't go back. I wish you the best for your journey in weight loss and in life.

Cheers,
Stephen Guise

More From Stephen

Check out **minihabits.com** for additional *Mini Habits for Weight Loss* content, tools, and resources!

Mini Habits
If you haven't yet, I strongly recommend you read my first book, *Mini Habits*. Although you don't need to read *Mini Habits* to benefit from *Mini Habits for Weight Loss*, it will give you more of the nuts and bolts of the original mini habits strategy.

Based on the science, *Mini Habits* is arguably the most effective habit formation strategy in the world. And, based on reviews, it's arguably the most loved and the most successful! Many lives have been transformed as a result of adopting the mini habits strategy. It can change your life too!

Mini Habits book: **http://amazon.com/dp/B00HGKNBDK**

Mini Habit Mastery
If you prefer video and want to learn the mini habits concept, you can take the Mini Habit Mastery Video Course. Use coupon code "MHWL55" for an exclusive *Mini Habits for Weight Loss* discount. Mini Habit Mastery is among the world's most popular habit courses, with over 9,000 students.

Mini Habit Mastery HD Video Course: **https://www.udemy.com/mini-habit-mastery/?couponCode=MHWL55**

How to Be an Imperfectionist
My second book applies *Mini Habits* to the problem of perfectionism. If you struggle with depression, fear, and inaction, this book has a lot to offer. It's the highest-rated product I've ever created.

How to Be an Imperfectionist book: **https://www.amazon.com/dp/B00UMG535Y**

Tuesday Messages
Every Tuesday, I write about smart life strategies and email them to subscribers. People have told me this content is life-changing. When you sign up, you can look through the archives of previous messages of interest. These are exclusive to subscribers and free. Also, signing up means you'll get to know when my next book or course is available.

Tuesday email sign-up: **http://stephenguise.com/subscribe/**

Thank You

Thank you so much for reading *Mini Habits for Weight Loss*. I hope you enjoyed it.

If you believe this book shares an important message, please leave a review on Amazon. Reviews (in quantity and in rating) are the main metric people use to judge a book's content. If you make progress, please come back and tell other readers (and me) about it!

Every single review has a huge impact on others' willingness to read a book, and if this strategy changes your life, you can change someone else's life by spreading the word. The impact and reach of this book is up to you. *Mini Habits* is proof of this. Because readers have reviewed and shared it, it is now read all over the world! Will you help me spread the message of *Mini Habits for Weight Loss*? The world needs to hear it.

Bonus content: **http://minihabits.com**
Contact Stephen: **sguise@deepexistence.com**

References

[1] Merriam-Webster.com. Retrieved 26 August 2016, from http://www.merriam-webster.com/dictionary/diet

[2] "The cycled animals required more than twice the time (21 vs. 46 days) to lose the same amount of weight during the second restriction compared to the first (food efficiency was increased 142%). One-third the time (10 vs. 29 days) was required to regain weight in the second refeeding. Food intake increased 25% and efficiency 52% in the second refeeding. The difference did not appear to be due to age, as efficiency decreased slightly over time in the age-matched Obese Controls while it increased significantly in the cycled animals."

Brownell, K., Greenwood, M., Stellar, E., & Shrager, E. (1986). *The effects of repeated cycles of weight loss and regain in rats.* Physiology & Behavior, 38(4), 459-464. http://dx.doi.org/10.1016/0031-9384(86)90411-7

[3] Bjorntorp, P., & Yang, M. U. (1982). *Refeeding after fasting in the rat: Effects on body composition and food efficiency.* Am J Clin Nutr 36: 444-449.

Walks, D., Lavau, M, Presta, E., Yang, M. U., & Bjorntorp, P. (1983). *Refeeding after fasting in the rat: Effects of dietary-induced obesity on energy balance regulation.* Am J Clin N, tr 37: 387-395.

Boyle, P. C., Storlien, L. H., Harper, A. E., & Keesey, R. E. (1981). *Oxygen consumption and locomotor activity during restricted feeding and realimentation.* Am J Physiol 241: R392-R387.

Boyle, P., Storlien, L., & Keesey, R. (1978). *Increased efficiency of food utilization following weight loss.* Physiology & Behavior, 21(2), 261-264. http://dx.doi.org/10.1016/0031-9384(78)90050-1

Levitsky, D., Faust, I., & Glassman, M. (1976). *The ingestion of food and the recovery of body weight following fasting in the naive rat.* Physiology & Behavior, 17(4), 575-580. http://dx.doi.org/10.1016/0031-9384(76)90154-2

Robinson, D., Hodgson, D., Bradford, G., Robb, J., & Peterson, D. (1975). *Effects of dietary restriction and fasting on the body composition of normal and genetically obese mice.* J Animal Science, 40(6), 1058. http://dx.doi.org/10.2527/jas1975.4061058x

Rolls, B., Rowe, E., & Turner, R. (1980). *Persistent obesity in rats following a period of consumption of a mixed, high energy diet.* J Physiology, 298(1), 415-427. http://dx.doi.org/10.1113/jphysiol.1980.sp013091

[4] Mann, T., Tomiyama, A., Westling, E., Lew, A., Samuels, B., & Chatman, J. (2007). *Medicare's search for effective obesity treatments: Diets are not the answer.* American Psychologist, 62(3), 220. Retrieved from http://psycnet.apa.org/index.cfm?fa=search.displayRecord&uid=2007-04834-008#

[5] Field, A., Austin, S., Taylor, C., Malspeis, S., Rosner, B., & Rockett, H., et al. (2003). *Relation between dieting and weight change among preadolescents and adolescents.* Pediatrics, 112(4), 900-906. Retrieved from http://pediatrics.aappublications.org/content/112/4/900

[6] Pietiläinen K. H. e. (2016). *Does dieting make you fat? A twin study.* PubMed - NCBI. Ncbi.nlm.nih.gov. Retrieved 26 August 2016, from https://www.ncbi.nlm.nih.gov/pubmed/21829159

[7] Tucker, T. (2006). *The great starvation experiment: the heroic men who starved so that millions could live.* New York: Free Press.

[8] Taubes, G. (2016). *Diet advice that ignores hunger.* Nytimes.com. Retrieved 26 August 2016, from http://www.nytimes.com/2015/08/30/opinion/diet-advice-that-ignores-hunger.html?_r=0

[9] Callahan, M. (2016). *The brutal secrets behind "The Biggest Loser".* Nypost.com. Retrieved 26 August 2016, from http://nypost.com/2015/01/18/contestant-reveals-the-brutal-secrets-of-the-biggest-loser/

[10] Fothergill, E., Guo, J., Howard, L., Kerns, J., Knuth, N., & Brychta, R., et al. (2016). *Persistent metabolic adaptation 6 years after "The Biggest Loser" competition.* Obesity, 24(8), 1612-1619. http://dx.doi.org/10.1002/oby.21538

[11] Mann, T., Tomiyama, A., Westling, E., Lew, A., Samuels, B., & Chatman, J. (2007). *Medicare's search for effective obesity treatments: Diets are not the answer.* American Psychologist, 62(3), 220. p. 222 Retrieved from http://psycnet.apa.org/

index.cfm?fa=search.displayRecord&uid=2007-04834-008#

[12] Howard BV, et al. (2006). *Low-fat dietary pattern and weight change over 7 years: The Women's Health Initiative Dietary Modification Trial.* Obstetrics & Gynecology, 107(4), 949. http://dx.doi.org/10.1097/01.aog.0000203661.68762.62

[13] Bailor, J. (2013). *The calorie myth.* Harper Wave.

[14] Hu, T., Mills, K., Yao, L., Demanelis, K., Eloustaz, M., & Yancy, W., et al. (2012). *Effects of low-carbohydrate diets versus low-fat diets on metabolic risk factors: A meta-analysis of randomized controlled clinical trials.* Am J Epidemiology, 176(suppl 7), S44-S54. http://dx.doi.org/10.1093/aje/kws264

[15] Hall, K. (2015). *Prescribing low-fat diets: Useless for long-term weight loss?* The Lancet Diabetes & Endocrinology, 3(12), 920-921. http://dx.doi.org/10.1016/s2213-8587(15)00413-1

[16] Lutes, L., Winett, R., Barger, S., Wojcik, J., Herbert, W., Nickols-Richardson, S., & Anderson, E. (2008). *Small changes in nutrition and physical activity promote weight loss and maintenance: 3-month evidence from the ASPIRE Randomized Trial.* Annals of Behavioral Medicine, 35(3), 351-357. http://dx.doi.org/10.1007/s12160-008-9033-z

[17] Gorin, A., Phelan, S., Wing, R., & Hill, J. (2003). *Promoting long-term weight control: Does dieting consistency matter?* Int J Obes Relat Metab Disord. http://dx.doi.org/10.1038/sj.ijo.0802550

[18] The 21 days idea came from the surgeon Maxwell Maltz, who observed it took a minimum of 21 days for amputees to get used to their new condition. It's no basis for making sweeping declarations on all human habit formation.

[19] Lally, P., van Jaarsveld, C., Potts, H., & Wardle, J. (2010). *How are habits formed: Modelling habit formation in the real world.* Eur J Social Psychology, 40(6), 998-1009. Retrieved from http://onlinelibrary.wiley.com/doi/10.1002/ejsp.674/abstract

[20] Norcross, J., Mrykalo, M., & Blagys, M. (2002). *Auld lang syne: Success predictors, change processes, and self-reported outcomes of New Year's resolvers and nonresolvers.* J Clinical Psychology, 58(4), 397-405. http://dx.doi.org/10.1002/jclp.1151

[21] Motivation is one of the top five most popular categories in nonfiction books, according to Amazon sales data.

[22] Kahneman, D. (2011-10-25). *Thinking, Fast and Slow* (p. 62). Farrar, Straus and Giroux. Kindle Edition.

[23] Kell, J. (2016). *Diet industry struggles as consumers eat more fresh food.* Fortune.com. Retrieved 26 August 2016, from

http://fortune.com/2015/05/22/lean-times-for-the-diet-industry/

[24] Some people intuitively realize the incongruence of "not enough desire" and "voluntarily suffering while paying $64 billion." They think if motivation isn't the problem, we just haven't found the right diet yet. But the equation itself is flawed, because "wanting it enough" and finding "the right diet" are not the crux of successful weight loss.

[25] Hagger, M., Wood, C., Stiff, C., & Chatzisarantis, N. (2010). *Ego depletion and the strength model of self-control: A meta-analysis.* Psychological Bulletin, 136(4), 495-525. http://dx.doi.org/10.1037/a0019486

[26] Researchers in the meta-analysis conducted at the University of Miami state: "Given the overall picture provided by our analyses, we conclude that the meta-analytic evidence does not support the proposition (and popular belief) that self-control functions as if it relies on a limited resource, at least when measured as it typically is in the laboratory. We encourage scientists and nonscientists alike to seriously consider other theories of when and why self-control might fail."[1]

Carter, et al. (2015). *Supplemental material for a series of meta-analytic tests of the depletion effect: Self-control does not seem to rely on a limited resource.* J Experimental Psychology: General. http://dx.doi.org/10.1037/xge0000083.supp

[27] Neal, D., Wood, W., & Quinn, J. (2006). *Habits—a repeat performance.* Current Directions in Psychological Science, 15(4), 198-202. http://dx.doi.org/10.1111/j.1467-8721.2006.00435.x

[28] Rehrer, C., Karimpour-Fard, A., Hernandez, T., Law, C., Stob, N., Hunter, L., & Eckel, R. (2012). *Regional differences in subcutaneous adipose tissue gene expression.* Obesity, 20(11), 2168-2173. http://dx.doi.org/10.1038/oby.2012.117

[29] Ryan, K., Woods, S., & Seeley, R. (2012). *Central nervous system mechanisms linking the consumption of palatable high-fat diets to the defense of greater adiposity.* Cell Metabolism, 15(2), 137-149. http://dx.doi.org/10.1016/j.cmet.2011.12.013

Jeanrenaud, B., (1997). *Central nervous system and body weight regulation.* PubMed - NCBI . Ncbi.nlm.nih.gov. Retrieved 30 August 2016, from https://www.ncbi.nlm.nih.gov/pubmed/9239233

[30] *Plastic surgery statistics show new consumer trends* | ASPS. (2016). Plasticsurgery.org. Retrieved 30 August 2016, from

http://www.plasticsurgery.org/news/2015/plastic-surgery-statistics-show-new-consumer-trends.html

[31] Weigle, D. (1994). *Appetite and the regulation of body composition*. The FASEB Journal, 8(3), 302-310. Retrieved from http://www.fasebj.org/content/8/3/302.long

[32] Kolata, G. (2016). *Study finds that fat cells die and are replaced*. Nytimes.com. Retrieved 30 August 2016, from http://www.nytimes.com/2008/05/05/health/research/05fat.html

[33] The idea behind intermittent fasting is that the fasting period doesn't last long enough to trigger this response from the body. One popular method is to eat in an eight-hour window every day. For example, you might eat all of your meals between 12 and 8 PM. How well it works is inconclusive and isn't addressed in this book.

[34] Attia, P. (2012). *Do calories matter?* The Eating Academy. Retrieved 30 August 2016, from http://eatingacademy.com/nutrition/do-calories-matter

[35] A gram is a measurement of mass, which tells us how much matter is in an object. Weight is how hard gravity pulls on an object's mass. Since we're all on earth, an object's weight and mass are going to be the same thing. On earth, the mass and weight of one egg is 50g. If you move an egg from earth to the moon, the mass will remain constant at 50g, but the weight will decrease to 8.3g.

I'll use the term weight because it's more commonly used and still accurate on earth. If you read this on the moon, please adjust accordingly (and invite me over for a basketball game so I can finally dunk on a 10-foot rim).

[36] Bailor, J. (2013). *The calorie myth*.

[37] St-Onge, M., & Jones, P. (2003). *Greater rise in fat oxidation with medium-chain triglyceride consumption relative to long-chain triglyceride is associated with lower initial body weight and greater loss of subcutaneous adipose tissue*. Int J Obes Relat Metab Disord, 27(12), 1565-1571. http://dx.doi.org/10.1038/sj.ijo.0802467

[38] Tucker, T. (2006). *The great starvation experiment*. New York: Free Press.

[39] Montmayeur, J., & Le Coutre, J. (2010). *Fat detection*. Boca Raton: CRC Press/Taylor & Francis.

[40] *Nutrition facts for your McDonald's meal*. (2016). FastFoodNutrition.org. Retrieved 30 August 2016, from http://fastfoodnutrition.org/calcresults?items[]=1901_1&items[]=1819_1&items[]=1888_1&rest=10

[41] Fardet, A. (2016). *Minimally processed foods are more satiating and less hyperglycemic than ultra-processed foods: A*

preliminary study with 98 ready-to-eat foods. Food Funct, 7(5), 2338-2346. http://dx.doi.org/10.1039/c6fo00107f

[42] Wal, J., Gupta, A., Khosla, P., & Dhurandhar, N. (2008). *Egg breakfast enhances weight loss*. Int J Obes Relat Metab Disord, 32(10), 1545-1551. http://dx.doi.org/10.1038/ijo.2008.130

[43] Urban, L., Lichtenstein, A., Gary, C., Fierstein, J., Equi, A., & Kussmaul, C., et al. (2013). *The energy content of restaurant foods without stated calorie information*. JAMA Internal Medicine, 173(14), 1292. http://dx.doi.org/10.1001/jamainternmed.2013.6163

[44] Holt, S. H. (1995). *A satiety index of common foods*. PubMed - NCBI. Ncbi.nlm.nih.gov. Retrieved 30 August 2016, from https://www.ncbi.nlm.nih.gov/pubmed/7498104

[45] Flynn, M., & Reinert, S. (2010). *Comparing an olive oil-enriched diet to a standard lower-fat diet for weight loss in breast cancer survivors: A pilot study*. J Women's Health, 19(6), 1155-1161. http://dx.doi.org/10.1089/jwh.2009.1759

[46] Das, U. (2001). *Is obesity an inflammatory condition?* Nutrition, 17(11-12), 953-966. http://dx.doi.org/10.1016/s0899-9007(01)00672-4

[47] Visser, M. (1999). *Elevated c-reactive protein levels in overweight and obese adults*. JAMA, 282(22), 2131. http://dx.doi.org/10.1001/jama.282.22.2131

[48] Das, 2001.

[49] Martin, S., Qasim, A., & Reilly, M. (2008). *Leptin resistance*. J Am College of Cardiology, 52(15), 1201-1210. http://dx.doi.org/10.1016/j.jacc.2008.05.060

[50] Fantuzzi, G., & Faggioni, R. (2000). *Leptin in the regulation of immunity, inflammation, and hematopoiesis*. PubMed - NCBI. Ncbi.nlm.nih.gov. Retrieved 31 August 2016, from https://www.ncbi.nlm.nih.gov/pubmed/11037963

[51] Chassaing, B., Koren, O., Goodrich, J., Poole, A., Srinivasan, S., Ley, R., & Gewirtz, A. (2015). *Dietary emulsifiers impact the mouse gut microbiota promoting colitis and metabolic syndrome*. Nature, 519(7541), 92-96. http://dx.doi.org/10.1038/nature14232

[52] Mozaffarian D., e. (2004). *Dietary intake of trans fatty acids and systemic inflammation in women*. PubMed - NCBI. Ncbi.nlm.nih.gov. Retrieved 31 August 2016, from https://www.ncbi.nlm.nih.gov/pubmed/15051604

[53] Kobylewski, S., & Jacobsen, M. (2012). Toxicology of food dyes. PubMed - NCBI. Ncbi.nlm.nih.gov. Retrieved 31 August 2016, from https://www.ncbi.nlm.nih.gov/pubmed/23026007

[54] Simopoulos, A. (2002). *The importance of the ratio of*

omega-6/omega-3 essential fatty acids. Biomedicine & Pharmacotherapy, 56(8), 365-379. http://dx.doi.org/10.1016/s0753-3322(02)00253-6

[55] Nakanishi, Y., Tsuneyama, K., Fujimoto, M., Salunga, T., Nomoto, K., & An, J., et al. (2008). *Monosodium glutamate (MSG): A villain and promoter of liver inflammation and dysplasia*. J of Autoimmunity, 30(1-2), 42-50. http://dx.doi.org/10.1016/j.jaut.2007.11.016

Just an anecdote about MSG: I ate at an Asian fusion restaurant one time, and about 20 minutes after the meal, which was delicious, I got a headache. Headaches are very rare for me, so I went back and asked the restaurant if my meal contained MSG, and sure enough, it was in the sauce. Mystery solved. I stopped eating there.

[56] Daniluk, J. (2012). *When food causes you pain.* CNN.com. Retrieved 31 August 2016, from http://www.cnn.com/2012/07/20/health/food-cause-pain-daniluk

[57] Elnahar, J. (2013). *Are vitamin supplements really bioavailable?* The Green Plate Special. Everydayhealth.com. Retrieved 31 August 2016, from http://www.everydayhealth.com/columns/jackie-arnett-green-plate-special/are-vitamin-supplements-really-bioavailable/

[58] Juul, F. & Hemmingsson, E. (2015). *Trends in consumption of ultra-processed foods and obesity in Sweden between 1960 and 2010*. Public Health Nutr, 18(17), 3096-3107. http://dx.doi.org/10.1017/s1368980015000506

[59] Martínez Steele, E., Baraldi, L., Louzada, M., Moubarac, J., Mozaffarian, D., & Monteiro, C. (2016). *Ultra-processed foods and added sugars in the US diet: Evidence from a nationally representative cross-sectional study*. BMJ Open, 6(3), e009892. http://dx.doi.org/10.1136/bmjopen-2015-009892

[60] *Trends in adult body-mass index in 200 countries from 1975 to 2014: A pooled analysis of 1,698 population-based measurement studies with 19.2 million participants* (2016). The Lancet, 387(10026), 1377-1396. http://dx.doi.org/10.1016/s0140-6736(16)30054-x

[61] Dutton, H. (1981). *History of the development of soy oil for edible uses*. J Am Oil Chem Soc, 58(3), 234-236. http://dx.doi.org/10.1007/bf02582347

[62] *Sugary drinks and obesity fact sheet* | The Nutrition Source | Harvard T. H. Chan School of Public Health (2016). Hsph.harvard.edu. Retrieved 31 August 2016, from https://www.hsph.harvard.edu/nutritionsource/sugary-drinks-fact-sheet/

[63] Maniam, J., Antoniadis, C., Youngson, N., Sinha, J., & Morris,

M. (2016). *Sugar consumption produces effects similar to early life stress exposure on hippocampal markers of neurogenesis and stress respons*e. Frontiers in Molecular Neurosci, 8. http://dx.doi.org/10.3389/fnmol.2015.00086

[64] Lustig, R., Mulligan, K., Noworolski, S., Tai, V., Wen, M., & Erkin-Cakmak, A., et al. (2015). *Isocaloric fructose restriction and metabolic improvement in children with obesity and metabolic syndrome.* Obesity, 24(2), 453-460. http://dx.doi.org/10.1002/oby.21371

[65] Nielsen, S., & Popkin, B. (2004). *Changes in beverage intake between 1977 and 2001.* Am J Preventive Medicine, 27(3), 205-210. http://dx.doi.org/10.1016/j.amepre.2004.05.005

[66] *Sugary drinks and obesity fact sheet* (2016).

[67] All four quotes are from: Parker, H. (2010). Princeton University. *A sweet problem: Princeton researchers find that high-fructose corn syrup prompts considerably more weight gain*. Princeton.edu. Retrieved 31 August 2016, from https://www.princeton.edu/main/news/archive/S26/91/22K07/

[68] Fagherazzi, G., Vilier, A., Saes Sartorelli, D., Lajous, M., Balkau, B., & Clavel-Chapelon, F. (2013). *Consumption of artificially and sugar-sweetened beverages and incident type 2 diabetes in the Etude Epidémiologique auprès des femmes de la Mutuelle Générale de l'Education Nationale - European Prospective Investigation into Cancer and Nutrition cohort.* Am J Clinical Nutrition, 97(3), 517-523. http://dx.doi.org/10.3945/ajcn.112.050997

[69] Lutsey, P., Steffen, L., & Stevens, J. (2008). *Dietary intake and the development of the metabolic syndrome: The atherosclerosis risk in communities study.* Circulation, 117(6), 754-761. http://dx.doi.org/10.1161/circulationaha.107.716159

[70] Suez, J., Korem, T., Zeevi, D., Zilberman-Schapira, G., Thaiss, C., & Maza, O., et al. (2014). *Artificial sweeteners induce glucose intolerance by altering the gut microbiota.* Nature. http://dx.doi.org/10.1038/nature13793

[71] Gottfried, J. (2011). *Neurobiology of sensation and reward.* CRC Press.

[72] Pierce, W., Heth, C., Owczarczyk, J., Russell, J., & Proctor, S. (2007). *Overeating by young obesity-prone and lean rats caused by tastes associated with low energy foods.* Obesity, 15(8), 1969-1979. http://dx.doi.org/10.1038/oby.2007.235

[73] Yang, Q. (2010). *Gain weight by "going diet?" Artificial sweeteners and the neurobiology of sugar cravings.* Neuroscience 2010. The Yale Journal of Biology and Medicine, 83(2), 101. Retrieved from https://www.ncbi.nlm.nih.gov/pmc/articles/PMC2892765/

[74] Yang, Q. *Gain weight by "going diet?"* (2010).

[75] Yang, Q. *Gain weight by "going diet?"* (2010).

[76] Liem, D., & Degraaf, C. (2004). *Sweet and sour preferences in young children and adults: Role of repeated exposure.* Physiology & Behavior, 83(3), 421-429. http://dx.doi.org/10.1016/j.physbeh.2004.08.028

[77] Fowler, S., Williams, K., Resendez, R., Hunt, K., Hazuda, H., & Stern, M. (2008). *Fueling the obesity epidemic? Artificially sweetened beverage use and long-term weight gain.* Obesity, 16(8), 1894-1900. http://dx.doi.org/10.1038/oby.2008.284

[78] Haribo Gummy Bear Product Page: www.amazon.com/Haribo-Gummy-Candy-Sugarless-5-Pound/dp/B000EVQWKC

[79] Murphy, L., & Coleman, A. (2012). *Xylitol toxicosis in dogs.* Veterinary Clinics of N America: Small Animal Practice, 42(2), 307-312. http://dx.doi.org/10.1016/j.cvsm.2011.12.003

[80] Schroder, K. (2010). *Effects of fruit consumption on body mass index and weight loss in a sample of overweight and obese dieters enrolled in a weight-loss intervention trial.* Nutrition, 26(7-8), 727-734. http://dx.doi.org/10.1016/j.nut.2009.08.009

[81] Bertoia, M., Rimm, E., Mukamal, K., Hu, F., Willett, W., & Cassidy, A. (2016). *Dietary flavonoid intake and weight maintenance: three prospective cohorts of 124,086 US men and women followed for up to 24 years.* BMJ, i17. http://dx.doi.org/10.1136/bmj.i17

[82] Bertoia, M., Mukamal, K., Cahill, L., Hou, T., Ludwig, D., & Mozaffarian, D., et al. (2016). *Changes in intake of fruits and vegetables and weight change in United States men and women followed for up to 24 years*: Analysis from Three Prospective Cohort Studies. Plos Med, 13(1), e1001956. http://dx.doi.org/10.1371/journal.pmed.1001956

[83] Lin, B. H., & Morrison, R. M. (2002). *Higher fruit consumption linked with lower body mass index.* Food Review, 25:28-32.

[84] Malik, V., Popkin, B., Bray, G., Despres, J., Willett, W., & Hu, F. (2010). *Sugar-sweetened beverages and risk of metabolic syndrome and type 2 diabetes: A meta-analysis.* Diabetes Care, 33(11), 2477-2483. http://dx.doi.org/10.2337/dc10-1079 Fagherazzi, G., et al. (2013).

[85] Muraki, I., Imamura, F., Manson, J., Hu, F., Willett, W., van Dam, R., & Sun, Q. (2013). *Fruit consumption and risk of type 2 diabetes: Results from three prospective longitudinal cohort studies.* BMJ, 347(aug28 1), f5001-f5001. http://dx.doi.org/10.1136/bmj.f5001

[86] Howard Perlman, U. (2016). *Water properties: The water in*

you. Water Science School. Water.usgs.gov. Retrieved 31 August 2016, from http://water.usgs.gov/edu/propertyyou.html

[87] Flood-Obbagy, J., & Rolls, B. (2009). *The effect of fruit in different forms on energy intake and satiety at a meal*. Appetite, 52(2), 416-422. http://dx.doi.org/10.1016/j.appet.2008.12.001

[88] Kaplan, K. (2014). *At least Americans aspire to be healthy eaters* .... LA Times. Retrieved 5 October 2016, from http://articles.latimes.com/2011/jan/04/news/la-heb-healthy-eating-survey-20100104

[89] Martínez Steele, E., et al. (2016).

[90] Dreher, M., & Davenport, A. (2013). *Hass avocado composition and potential health effects*. Critical Reviews in Food Sci & Nutrition, 53(7), 738-750. http://dx.doi.org/10.1080/10408398.2011.556759

[91] *DMU research on 'healthiest' cooking oils revealed on BBC's Trust Me, I'm a Doctor* (2016). De Montfort University. Retrieved 5 October 2016, from https://www.dmu.ac.uk/about-dmu/news/2015/july/dmu-research-on-healthiest-cooking-oils-revealed-on-bbcs-trust-me,-im-a-doctor.aspx

[92] Katragadda, H., Fullana, A., Sidhu, S., & Carbonell-Barrachina, Á. (2010). *Emissions of volatile aldehydes from heated cooking oils*. Food Chemistry, 120(1), 59-65. http://dx.doi.org/10.1016/j.foodchem.2009.09.070

[93] Zemel, M., Thompson, W., Milstead, A., Morris, K., & Campbell, P. (2004). *Calcium and dairy acceleration of weight and fat loss during energy restriction in obese adults*. Obesity Research, 12(4), 582-590. http://dx.doi.org/10.1038/oby.2004.67

[94] Rosell, M., Håkansson, N., & Wolk, A. (2006). *Association between dairy food consumption and weight change over 9 y in 19,352 perimenopausal women*. Am J of Clinical Nutrition, 84(6), 1481-1488. Retrieved from http://ajcn.nutrition.org/content/84/6/1481.full

[95] Rautiainen, S., Wang, L., Lee, I., Manson, J., Buring, J., & Sesso, H. (2016). *Dairy consumption in association with weight change and risk of becoming overweight or obese in middle-aged and older women: a prospective cohort study*. Am J Clinical Nutrition, 103(4), 979-988. http://dx.doi.org/10.3945/ajcn.115.118406

[96] Holmberg, S., & Thelin, A. (2013). *High dairy fat intake related to less central obesity: A male cohort study with 12 years' follow-up*. Scandinavian J Primary Health Care, 31(2), 89-94. http://dx.doi.org/10.3109/02813432.2012.757070

[97] Scharf, R., Demmer, R., & DeBoer, M. (2013). *Longitudinal*

evaluation of milk type consumed and weight status in preschoolers. Archives of Disease in Childhood, 98(5), 335-340. http://dx.doi.org/10.1136/archdischild-2012-302941

[98] *Fattening pigs for market* (1930). Ir.library.oregonstate.edu. Retrieved 5 October 2016, from https:// ir.library.oregonstate.edu/xmlui/bitstream/handle/1957/14694/ StationBulletin269.pdf?sequence=1

[99] Carwile, J., & Michels, K. (2011). *Urinary bisphenol A and obesity*: NHANES 2003–2006. Environmental Research, 111(6), 825-830. http://dx.doi.org/10.1016/j.envres.2011.05.014

Xu, X., Tan, L., Himi, T., Sadamatsu, M., Tsutsumi, S., Akaike, M., & Kato, N. (2011). *Changed preference for sweet taste in adulthood induced by perinatal exposure to bisphenol A: A probable link to overweight and obesity*. Neurotoxicology and Teratology, 33(4), 458-463. http://dx.doi.org/10.1016/j.ntt. 2011.06.002

[100] Wang, T., Li, M., Chen, B., Xu, M., Xu, Y., & Huang, Y., et al. (2012). *Urinary bisphenol A (BPA) concentration associates with obesity and insulin resistance*. J of Clinical Endocrinology & Metabolism, 97(2), E223-E227. http://dx.doi.org/10.1210/jc. 2011-1989

[101] Pupo, M., Pisano, A., Lappano, R., Santolla, M., De Francesco, E., & Abonante, S., et al. (2012). *Bisphenol A induces gene expression changes and proliferative effects through GPER in breast cancer cells and cancer-associated fibroblasts*. Environmental Health Perspectives, 120(8), 1177-1182. http://dx.doi.org/10.1289/ehp.1104526

Prins, G., Hu, W., Shi, G., Hu, D., Majumdar, S., & Li, G., et al. (2014). *Bisphenol A promotes human prostate stem-progenitor cell self-renewal and increases in vivo carcinogenesis in human prostate epithelium*. Endocrinology, 155(3), 805-817. http:// dx.doi.org/10.1210/en.2013-1955

[102] Stern, V. (2015). *Mythbusters: Does this cause cancer?* Medscape. Retrieved 5 October 2016, from http:// www.medscape.com/viewarticle/840559

[103] *Consuming canned soup linked to greatly elevated levels of the chemical BPA* (2011). Harvard. Retrieved 5 October 2016, from https://www.hsph.harvard.edu/news/press-releases/ canned-soup-bpa/

[104] *Drink water to curb weight gain? Clinical trial confirms effectiveness of simple appetite control method* (2010). ScienceDaily. Retrieved 5 October 2016, from https:// www.sciencedaily.com/releases/2010/08/100823142929.htm

[105] Boschmann, M., Steiniger, J., Hille, U., Tank, J., Adams, F., & Sharma, A., et al. (2003). *Water-induced thermogenesis*. J of Clinical Endocrinology & Metabolism, 88(12), 6015-6019. http://dx.doi.org/10.1210/jc.2003-030780

[106] Nagao, T., et al. (2005). *Ingestion of a tea rich in catechins leads to a reduction in body fat and malondialdehyde-modified LDL in men*. PubMed - NCBI. Ncbi.nlm.nih.gov. Retrieved 5 October 2016, from https://www.ncbi.nlm.nih.gov/pubmed/15640470

Zhang, Y., Yu, Y., Li, X., Meguro, S., Hayashi, S., & Katashima, M., et al. (2012). *Effects of catechin-enriched green tea beverage on visceral fat loss in adults with a high proportion of visceral fat: A double-blind, placebo-controlled, randomized trial*. J of Functional Foods, 4(1), 315-322. http://dx.doi.org/10.1016/j.jff.2011.12.010

[107] Grønbæk, M. (2000). *Type of alcohol consumed and mortality from all causes, coronary heart disease, and cancer*. Annals of Internal Medicine, 133(6), 411. http://dx.doi.org/10.7326/0003-4819-133-6-200009190-00008

[108] Wang, L. (2010). *Alcohol consumption, weight gain, and risk of becoming overweight in middle-aged and older women*. Archives of Internal Medicine, 170(5), 453. http://dx.doi.org/10.1001/archinternmed.2009.527

[109] Phillips, R. (2015). *WSU scientists turn white fat into obesity-fighting beige fat | WSU News | Washington State University*. Retrieved 5 October 2016, from https://news.wsu.edu/2015/06/18/wsu-scientists-turn-white-fat-into-obesity-fighting-beige-fat/

[110] Loyola University Health System (2015). *Exercise alone does not help in losing weight*. ScienceDaily. Retrieved 31 August 2016, from https://www.sciencedaily.com/releases/2015/08/150817142140.htm

[111] Johns, D., Hartmann-Boyce, J., Jebb, S., & Aveyard, P. (2014). *Diet or exercise interventions vs combined behavioral weight management programs: A systematic review and meta-analysis of direct comparisons*. J of Academy of Nutrition and Dietetics, 114(10), 1557-1568. http://dx.doi.org/10.1016/j.jand.2014.07.005

[112] *National weight control registry facts* (2016). Nwcr.ws. Retrieved 3 September 2016, from http://nwcr.ws/Research/default.htm

[113] Hankinson, A., Daviglus, M., Bouchard, C., Carnethon, M., Lewis, C., & Schreiner, P., et al. (2010). *Maintaining a high physical activity level over 20 years and weight gain*. JAMA,

304(23), 2603. http://dx.doi.org/10.1001/jama.2010.1843
[114] Nelson, R., Horowitz, J., Holleman, R., Swartz, A., Strath, S., Kriska, A., & Richardson, C. (2013). *Daily physical activity predicts degree of insulin resistance: a cross-sectional observational study using the 2003–2004 National Health and Nutrition Examination Survey.* Int J Behav Nutr Phys Act, 10(1), 10. http://dx.doi.org/10.1186/1479-5868-10-10

Borghouts, L., & Keizer, H. (2000). *Exercise and insulin sensitivity: A review.* International J of Sports Medicine, 21(1), 1-12. http://dx.doi.org/10.1055/s-2000-8847
[115] Ross, R., & Janssen, I. (1999). *Is abdominal fat preferentially reduced in response to exercise-induced weight loss?* Medicine & Science in Sports & Exercise, 31(Supplement 1), S568. http://dx.doi.org/10.1097/00005768-199911001-00014
[116] Melanson, E., MacLean, P., & Hill, J. (2009). *Exercise improves fat metabolism in muscle but does not increase 24-h fat oxidation.* Exercise and Sport Sciences Reviews, 37(2), 93-101. http://dx.doi.org/10.1097/jes.0b013e31819c2f0b
[117] Nedeltcheva, A., Kilkus, J., Imperial, J., Schoeller, D., & Penev, P. (2010). *Insufficient sleep undermines dietary efforts to reduce adiposity.* Annals of Internal Medicine, 153(7), 435. http://dx.doi.org/10.7326/0003-4819-153-7-201010050-00006
[118] Note: Throughout this book, I state that calories don't matter, but that's only for lasting weight loss. Since I reference studies that use caloric input as a control, it's important to understand that calorie intake is a viable short-term predictor of weight impact. Calorie intake is the most important short-term factor for weight change—evidenced by the fact you can starve yourself and lose weight rapidly—but it's foolish as an eating guide in the long term. Calorie deficits and surpluses are a byproduct of your eating habits, movement habits, and food factors like satiety, calorie density, and nutrition, all of which affect your appetite and metabolic function over the long term.
[119] Taheri, S., Lin, L., Austin, D., Young, T., & Mignot, E. (2004). *Short sleep duration is associated with reduced leptin, elevated ghrelin, and increased Body Mass Index.* Plos Med, 1(3), e62. http://dx.doi.org/10.1371/journal.pmed.0010062
[120] Werle, C., Wansink, B., & Payne, C. (2015) *Is it fun or exercise? The framing of physical activity biases subsequent snacking.* SSRN Electronic Journal. http://dx.doi.org/10.2139/ssrn.2442383
[121] King, A., Castro, C., Buman, M., Hekler, E., Urizar, G., & Ahn, D. (2013). *Behavioral impacts of sequentially versus*

simultaneously delivered dietary plus physical activity interventions: the CALM Trial. Annals of Behavioral Medicine, 46(2), 157-168. http://dx.doi.org/10.1007/s12160-013-9501-y

[122] Martínez Steele, E., et al. (2016).

[123] Inspired by a quote from Derek Sivers (sivers.org).

[124] Dalle Grave, R., Calugi, S., Molinari, E., Petroni, M., Bondi, M., Compare, A., & Marchesini, G. (2005). *Weight loss expectations in obese patients and treatment attrition: An observational multicenter study*. Obesity Research, 13(11), 1961-1969. http://dx.doi.org/10.1038/oby.2005.241

[125] Patrick, V., & Hagtvedt, H. (2012). *"I don't" versus "I can't": When empowered refusal motivates goal-directed behavior*. J Consum Res, 39(2), 371-381. http://dx.doi.org/10.1086/663212

[126] Patrick, V., & Hagtvedt, H. (2012).

[127] Bertoia, M., et al. (2016). *Changes in intake of fruits and vegetables and weight change in United States men and women followed for up to 24 years.*

[128] Bennett, G., Foley, P., Levine, E., Whiteley, J., Askew, S., & Steinberg, D., et al. (2013). *Behavioral treatment for weight gain prevention among Black women in primary care practice*. JAMA Internal Medicine, 173(19), 1770. http://dx.doi.org/10.1001/jamainternmed.2013.9263

[129] Fowler, S., Williams, K., Resendez, R., Hunt, K., Hazuda, H., & Stern, M. (2008). *Fueling the obesity epidemic? Artificially sweetened beverage use and long-term weight gain*. Obesity, 16(8), 1894-1900. http://dx.doi.org/10.1038/oby.2008.284

[130] Laska, M., Murray, D., Lytle, L., & Harnack, L. (2011). *Longitudinal associations between key dietary behaviors and weight gain over time: Transitions through the adolescent years*. Obesity, 20(1), 118-125. http://dx.doi.org/10.1038/oby.2011.179

[131] Dalle Grave, R., et al., (2005).

[132] Burgo, J. (2013). *The difference between guilt and shame*. Psychology Today. Retrieved 18 October 2016, from https://www.psychologytoday.com/blog/shame/201305/the-difference-between-guilt-and-shame

[133] Kolata, G. (2016). *After 'The Biggest Loser,' their bodies fought to regain weight*. Nytimes.com. Retrieved 6 October 2016, from http://www.nytimes.com/2016/05/02/health/biggest-loser-weight-loss.html

[134] Frankel, et al. (2011). *Evaluation of extra-virgin olive oil sold in California*. UCDavis.edu. Retrieved 6 October 2016, from http://olivecenter.ucdavis.edu/research/files/

report041211finalreduced.pdf

[135] *The best extra-virgin olive oil.* Consumer Reports Magazine. (2012). Consumerreports.org. Retrieved 6 October 2016, from http://www.consumerreports.org/cro/magazine/2012/09/how-to-find-the-best-extra-virgin-olive-oil/index.htm

[136] Morris, M., Na, E., & Johnson, A. (2008). *Salt craving: The psychobiology of pathogenic sodium intake.* Physiology & Behavior, 94(5), 709-721. http://dx.doi.org/10.1016/j.physbeh.2008.04.008

[137] www.aol.com/food/three-quickest-ways-microwave-eggs/

[138] Vander Wal, J., Marth, J., Khosla, P., Jen, K., & Dhurandhar, N. (2005). *Short-term effect of eggs on satiety in overweight and obese subjects.* J Am College of Nutrition, 24(6), 510-515. http://dx.doi.org/10.1080/07315724.2005.10719497

[139] Type "water infuser" into Amazon's search bar. Even if you don't buy from Amazon, it's a great place to see reviews.

[140] Li, J., Zhang, N., Hu, L., Li, Z., Li, R., Li, C., & Wang, S. (2011). *Improvement in chewing activity reduces energy intake in one meal and modulates plasma gut hormone concentrations in obese and lean young Chinese men.* Am J Clinical Nutrition, 94(3), 709-716. http://dx.doi.org/10.3945/ajcn.111.015164

[141] Vartanian, L., & Novak, S. (2010). *Internalized societal attitudes moderate the impact of weight stigma on avoidance of exercise.* Obesity, 19(4), 757-762. http://dx.doi.org/10.1038/oby.2010.234

[142] Hoffman, B., & Blumenthal, J. (2012). *Is exercise a viable treatment for depression?* ACSM's Health & Fitness Journal, 16(4), 14. Retrieved from https://www.ncbi.nlm.nih.gov/pmc/articles/PMC3674785/

[143] Matthews, C., Chen, K., Freedson, P., Buchowski, M., Beech, B., Pate, R., & Troiano, R. (2008). *Amount of time spent in sedentary behaviors in the United States, 2003-2004.* Am J Epidemiology, 167(7), 875-881. http://dx.doi.org/10.1093/aje/kwm390

[144] Boscia, T. (2014). *Study: prolonged sitting jeopardizes older women's health* | Cornell Chronicle. News.cornell.edu. Retrieved 6 October 2016, from http://www.news.cornell.edu/stories/2014/01/study-prolonged-sitting-jeopardizes-older-women-s-health

[145] Patel, A., Bernstein, L., Deka, A., Feigelson, H., Campbell, P., & Gapstur, S., et al. (2010). *Leisure time spent sitting in relation to total mortality in a prospective cohort of US adults.* Am J Epidemiology, 172(4), 419-429. http://dx.doi.org/10.1093/aje/kwq155

[146] van der Ploeg, H. (2012). *Sitting time and all-cause mortality risk in 222,497 Australian adults*. Archives of Internal Medicine, 172(6), 494. http://dx.doi.org/10.1001/archinternmed.2011.2174

[147] Levine, J. (2005). *Interindividual variation in posture allocation: Possible role in human obesity*. Science, 307(5709), 584-586. http://dx.doi.org/10.1126/science.1106561

[148] *Calorie burner: How much better is standing up than sitting?* (2013). BBC News. Retrieved 6 October 2016, from http://www.bbc.com/news/magazine-24532996

[149] Levine, J. (2010). *James Levine, M.D., Ph.D. - Transform 2010 - Mayo Clinic*. YouTube. Retrieved 6 October 2016, from https://www.youtube.com/watch?v=S6eIvxqaezE

[150] Dahl, M. (2015). *I am training for a marathon. So why am I getting fat?* Science of Us. Retrieved 6 October 2016, from http://nymag.com/scienceofus/2015/10/on-the-mysteries-of-marathon-weight-gain.html

[151] Boutcher, S. (2011). *High-intensity intermittent exercise and fat loss*. J Obesity, 2011, 1-10. http://dx.doi.org/10.1155/2011/868305

[152] Tremblay, A., Simoneau, J., & Bouchard, C. (1994). *Impact of exercise intensity on body fatness and skeletal muscle metabolism*. Metabolism, 43(7), 814-818. http://dx.doi.org/10.1016/0026-0495(94)90259-3

[153] "The mean estimated total energy cost of the ET program was 120.4 MJ, whereas the corresponding value for the HIIT program was 57.9 MJ." (Tremblay, et al., 1994)

[154] Trapp, E., Chisholm, D., Freund, J., & Boutcher, S. (2008). *The effects of high-intensity intermittent exercise training on fat loss and fasting insulin levels of young women*. International J Obesity, 32(4), 684-691. http://dx.doi.org/10.1038/sj.ijo.0803781

[155] Macpherson, R., Hazell, T., Olver, T., Paterson, D., & Lemon, P. (2011). *Run sprint interval training improves aerobic performance but not maximal cardiac output*. Medicine & Science in Sports & Exercise, 43(1), 115-122. http://dx.doi.org/10.1249/mss.0b013e3181e5eacd

[156] Sim, A., Wallman, K., Fairchild, T., & Guelfi, K. (2013). *High-intensity intermittent exercise attenuates ad-libitum energy intake*. International J Obesity, 38(3), 417-422. http://dx.doi.org/10.1038/ijo.2013.102

[157] Seventeen men were tested in four different exercise scenarios on different days. One day, the men rested for 30 minutes. Another day, they rode an exercise bike for 30

minutes at 65% of their aerobic capacity (which is said to be the optimal "fat burn zone"). A third session did one minute at 100% capacity, followed by four minutes of gentle pedaling for 30 minutes. The final session was a calculated 170% of their capacity for just 15 seconds, followed by gentle pedaling for a minute, repeated for 30 minutes. After each session, they were given bland, slightly sweetened porridge to eat. On the interval session days, they consumed significantly less than they did on the resting and moderate training days (the 15-second interval resulted in the least amount consumed, suggesting an inverse relationship between intensity and appetite). The results appeared to be due to chemical changes induced by exercise.

The men's blood was tested, and showed lower ghrelin, higher blood lactate, and higher blood sugar on interval training days, all of which have been shown to lessen appetite. Surprisingly, this effect carried over to the next day and they consumed fewer calories in the following 24 hours. This is in stark contrast to the resting and moderate exercise days, in which the men voraciously consumed the porridge.

This was a short and limited study that was only done for young overweight males, but it's promising nonetheless when considered alongside the other data we have on high-intensity exercise. Anecdotally, it completely matches my experience. When I was a teenager, I would play full-court basketball for up to six hours straight, and despite not eating at all during that time and desperately needing to eat after using so much energy, I would come home and be unable to eat for at least another hour or two. It would completely shut down my appetite!

[158] Benito, B., Gay-Jordi, G., Serrano-Mollar, A., Guasch, E., Shi, Y., & Tardif, J., et al. (2010). *Cardiac arrhythmogenic remodeling in a rat model of long-term intensive exercise training*. Circulation, 123(1), 13-22. http://dx.doi.org/10.1161/circulationaha.110.938282

Pappas, S. (2010). *Temporary heart damage may explain marathon deaths*. Live Science. Retrieved 18 October 2016, from http://www.livescience.com/10211-temporary-heart-damage-explain-marathon-deaths.html

[159] O'Keefe, J., Patil, H., Lavie, C., Magalski, A., Vogel, R., & McCullough, P. (2012). *Potential adverse cardiovascular effects from excessive endurance exercise*. Mayo Clinic Proceedings, 87(6), 587-595. http://dx.doi.org/10.1016/j.mayocp.2012.04.005

[160] Wilson, M., O'Hanlon, R., Prasad, S., Deighan, A., MacMillan, P., & Oxborough, D., et al. (2011). *Diverse patterns of myocardial fibrosis in lifelong, veteran endurance athletes*. J Applied Physiology, 110(6), 1622-1626. http://dx.doi.org/10.1152/japplphysiol.01280.2010

[161] Rognmo, O., Moholdt, T., Bakken, H., Hole, T., Molstad, P., & Myhr, N., et al. (2012). *Cardiovascular risk of high- versus moderate-intensity aerobic exercise in coronary heart disease patients*. Circulation, 126(12), 1436-1440. http://dx.doi.org/10.1161/circulationaha.112.123117

[162] Melanson, E., MacLean, P., & Hill, J. (2009). *Exercise improves fat metabolism in muscle but does not increase 24-h fat oxidation*. Exercise & Sport Sciences Reviews, 37(2), 93-101. http://dx.doi.org/10.1097/jes.0b013e31819c2f0b

[163] King, J., Wasse, L., Broom, D., & Stensel, D. (2010). *Influence of brisk walking on appetite, energy intake, and plasma acylated ghrelin*. Medicine & Science in Sports & Exercise, 42(3), 485-492. http://dx.doi.org/10.1249/mss.0b013e3181ba10c4

[164] *NWCR research findings*. (2016). The National Weight Control Registry. Retrieved 18 October 2016, from http://www.nwcr.ws/research/

[165] Willis, L., Slentz, C., Bateman, L., Shields, A., Piner, L., & Bales, C., et al. (2012). *Effects of aerobic and/or resistance training on body mass and fat mass in overweight or obese adults*. J Applied Physiology, 113(12), 1831-1837. http://dx.doi.org/10.1152/japplphysiol.01370.2011

[166] Lally, P., van Jaarsveld, C., Potts, H., & Wardle, J. (2010). *How are habits formed: Modelling habit formation in the real world*. European Journal of Social Psychology, 40(6), 998-1009. Retrieved from http://onlinelibrary.wiley.com/doi/10.1002/ejsp.674/abstract

[167] www.ewg.org/foodnews/list.php

[168] Benbrook, C., Butler, G., Latif, M., Leifert, C., & Davis, D. (2013). *Organic production enhances milk nutritional quality by shifting fatty acid composition: A United States–wide, 18-month study*. Plos ONE, 8(12), e82429. http://dx.doi.org/10.1371/journal.pone.0082429

[169] McGonigal, K. (2012). *The willpower instinct*. New York: Avery.

[170] Monteleone, P., Piscitelli, F., Scognamiglio, P., Monteleone, A., Canestrelli, B., Di Marzo, V., & Maj, M. (2012). *Hedonic eating is associated with increased peripheral levels of ghrelin and the endocannabinoid 2-arachidonoyl-glycerol in healthy humans: A pilot study*. J Clinical Endocrinology & Metabolism,

97(6), E917-E924. http://dx.doi.org/10.1210/jc.2011-3018

[171] Rao, M., Afshin, A., Singh, G., & Mozaffarian, D. (2013). *Do healthier foods and diet patterns cost more than less healthy options? A systematic review and meta-analysis.* BMJ Open, 3(12), e004277. http://dx.doi.org/10.1136/bmjopen-2013-004277

[172] Ogden CL, Kit BK, Carroll MD, Park S. *Consumption of sugar drinks in the United States, 2005–2008.* NCHS data brief, no 71. Hyattsville, MD: National Center for Health Statistics. 2011.

[173] Ricard, M. (2004). *The habits of happiness.* Ted.com. Retrieved 18 October 2016, from http://www.ted.com/talks/matthieu_ricard_on_the_habits_of_happiness.html

[174] Kell, J. (2016). *Soda consumption falls to 30-year low in the US.* Fortune. Retrieved 18 October 2016, from http://fortune.com/2016/03/29/soda-sales-drop-11th-year/

[175] Jones, J. (2010). *Holiday weight gain: A growing problem | November | 2010 | Texas Tech Today | TTU.* Today.ttu.edu. Retrieved 18 October 2016, from http://today.ttu.edu/posts/2010/11/holiday-weight-gain-a-growing-problem

Made in the USA
San Bernardino, CA
18 October 2017